A Nurse
in Action

993385550 6

WITHDRAWN
FOR SALE

Also by Evelyn Prentis

A Nurse in Time

A Nurse in Action

My Life as a Nurse in the Second World War

EVELYN PRENTIS

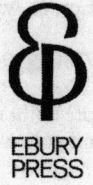

EBURY
PRESS

3 5 7 9 10 8 6 4 2

This edition published 2011 by Ebury Press, an imprint
of Ebury Publishing
A Random House Group company
First published in 1978 by Hutchinson & Co (Publishers) Ltd

Copyright © Evelyn Prentis 1978

Evelyn Prentis has asserted her right to be identified as the author of this
Work in accordance with the Copyright, Designs and Patents Act 1988

The Random House Group Limited Reg. No. 954009

Addresses for companies within the Random House Group can be
found at www.randomhouse.co.uk

A CIP catalogue record for this book is available from
the British Library

The Random House Group Limited supports the Forest Stewardship
Council® (FSC®), the leading international forest certification
organisation. All our titles that are printed on Greenpeace approved
FSC® certified paper carry the FSC® logo. Our paper procurement
policy can be found at www.randomhouse.co.uk/environment

Printed in the UK by CPI Cox & Wyman, Reading, RG1 8EX

ISBN 9780091941376

To buy books by your favourite authors and register for offers visit
www.randomhouse.co.uk

For Judith and Barbara
with love

Part One

Chapter One

I STOOD ON the mat in the Matron's office, feet shuffling nervously, palms sweating, exactly as I had stood on it so often since the day I started my training. It was a poor threadbare little mat, worn thin in the middle by the nervous shuffling of generations of nurses before me. The same shabby little mat I had sprawled headlong on, the morning I was summoned to the office for the first time. Missing the step and falling flat on my face had done nothing to make my debut into nursing a thing of joy. Then, as now, the Matron had looked at me coldly and was not amused. Then, as now, the fat Scottie dog at his post by the desk had bared his teeth contemptuously. Now as then I quailed before the look and shrank from the dog's bad breath. It seemed that nothing had changed. Nor ever would.

Yet changes there had been. I was no longer a probationer nurse, butterfly cap concealing my ears, anchored there hopefully by a dozen Kirby grips. I had passed my Finals, and was now a staff-nurse, entitled to wear a little bonnet of a cap held firmly in place by a length of tape and a pair of lacy bows. Only that morning I had read my name on the pass list, rushed across to my room, rescued the bows from the back of a drawer, ironed them by sitting on them then proudly put them on. Though I had worn them for such a short time their starched crispness was already chafing red weals beneath my chubby chin. They were still new enough to give me an exaggerated sense of my own importance.

The Matron quickly took away some of that importance. She glanced at the bows, raised her eyebrows and spoke. 'Good morning, Nurse,' she said. 'I see by your bows that you managed to pass your Finals.' There was a touch of ice and disbelief in her voice that suggested she was as astonished as I had been that I could ever have achieved such a miracle. It had taken some achieving. There had been things the oral examiners and I had failed to reach any agreement over, and several of the statements I had made on the written papers were open to debate. I left the examination centre gloomily certain that I would remain a probationer for ever. It was therefore not surprising that the Matron found it hard to believe that I could have blossomed overnight from a Kirby-gripped junior to a bow-bedecked staff-nurse. There was clearly etched on her mind an imprint of the laziness, slackness, inattention to detail, and total lack of aptitude for nursing that had brought me in disgrace to her office so many times during the past three years. Each of my sins, from the palest grey to the deepest black, had been remembered and recorded, ready to tell against me whenever I presented myself on the little mat, as they were doing now.

I remained stiffly silent, consoling myself with the thought that the reception I was getting would have been no warmer if I had been a born nurse – which I most certainly wasn't – a paragon of efficiency and a second coming of Florence Nightingale, all neatly packaged in my blue striped uniform. The Matron treated everybody with the same chilling aloofness. She was the Eternal Matron. Her bows were larger, lacier and starchier than any other bows in the hospital. They nestled confidently between her second and third chins and wobbled as she spoke. They were the metronome our hopes and fears were adjusted to. While they ticked over steadily we sweated less, as their tempo increased we oozed accordingly.

The Matron was the axis of our world, feared by the nurses from the highest to the lowest and held in awed respect by the most senior of the honorary consultants. While she sat at her desk, unmoved and largely unmoving, we felt safe in the knowledge that the hospital and all that therein was would go on revolving regardless of anything that went on in the world outside. We were soon to find that not even she could remain impervious to the things that were going on in the world in 1938.

Her bows started twitching again. They sank in anticipation as she opened her mouth and rose up sharply when she snapped out her censure.

'Your record over the last years has not been particularly outstanding, Nurse,' she said, then waited for me to agree with her. She didn't have long to wait. I had been brought up to respect my elders and fear my betters. There was not the remotest possibility of my disagreeing with her.

'Yes, Matron,' I agreed. 'No, Matron,' I amended hastily.

Her eyes slid over my apron, crumpled but clean, rested briefly on my collar, smooth but grubby, took in the bonnet and came to rest on the bows which by now had started to shrink into insignificance.

'I trust you will carry out your duties as a staff-nurse with greater assiduity than you employed while you were muddling through them as a probationer,' she said coldly, and paused to give me time to mull over assiduity. I mulled over it. Muddle I was familiar with. Assiduity I was not. I was no wiser after I had finished mulling than I was before.

'Yes, Matron, thank you, Matron,' I breathed gratefully, and left the office.

Over in the drab unfurnished room we called the library, which was the only place in the nurses' home where we were allowed to smoke and almost certainly the only room in the hospital where there was not a book in sight, Baker, Weldon, Davies and the Irish girl were already smoking. They had been by my side through the years of toil, stress and strain, getting far more fun out of it than any of us had ever expected to get when we started our training. They also had passed their Finals and done their shuffling on the Matron's mat and were celebrating the glorious victory over the enemy examiners with cheap cigarettes. Like me, they desperately needed nicotine to calm their Matron-shattered nerves.

I accepted a Woodbine from Baker and applied it to the glowing end of the Irish girl's Park Drive. It was the middle of the month and the last payday but a bygone memory and the next too far away to be more than a promise for the future. None of us could run to the more luxurious brands of cigarettes. There were those amongst us who could scarcely afford even the cheaper sort. Weldon was spending her thirty shillings a month salary almost as fast as she got it on fripperies for her bottom drawer, which meant that she was cadging fags off us long before payday, and Davies was blessed with a streak of Welsh prudence that drove her to the Post Office every month to deposit small sums against penury in her old age. I had no such streak. I was destined to penury from the start. Nor had I a bottom drawer to worry about. I was twenty-one and had already resigned myself to spinsterhood.

Weldon helped herself to my last de Reszke Minor, broke it in half and gave half to Davies.

'Well, what did she say to you?' she asked me, throwing the empty packet out of the window for a gardener to curse about when he had to bend his back to pick it up. She and Davies both knew that I would never have grudged them my last cigarette. Not at any rate while Baker had some left to share with me. From the start of our training they had been something special in the way of friends; eager with their advice whether I asked for it or not and offering support when I looked like sagging. Though we hadn't always seen eye to eye, they were the first to admit that it took all sorts to make a world and I was definitely a different sort from either them or Baker. I had none of the indefinable qualities which had turned them into born nurses but this had caused no permanent rifts in our friendship.

They may have sometimes been driven to criticize my wilder indiscretions but their criticisms had never been too destructive. Without them my training days would have been far less rewarding than they were.

I waited until we were all nicely lit up, then I told them how astonished the Matron was when she saw that I had passed my Finals. I gave them a lively demonstration of the gymnastics of her bows, and a run-through of the critical assessment she had made of my progress, paying special attention to the word 'assiduity'. When I had finished the demonstration and concluded the assessment Baker started to giggle. Baker was a happy, buxom girl, always able to see a silver gleam behind the most threatening cloud. This was to be a great asset to her when the clouds had grown so threatening that it was almost impossible to get even the smallest gleam out of them.

'My God,' she said. 'She must have it written down in front of her on a piece of paper. She said exactly the same to me.' 'And to me,' echoed the others. This didn't surprise me at all. The speech had sounded much too set to be a one-off. We stood for a moment thinking about it then Davies looked round at us. 'As a matter of interest,' she said in a serious way, 'what exactly does assiduity mean?' Davies said most things in a serious way. She was a very serious girl. She lacked the more relaxed approach to life that made living so bearable for Baker. Clouds already tinged with grey became ever more grey for Davies.

The Irish girl allowed a ring of smoke to curl to the grimy ceiling before she came up with her definition of the word 'assiduity'. When she gave it to us it was an extremely Irish definition. 'It sounds as though it should have something to do with acid,' she said, watching the smoke rise like incense, 'as in urine testing and litmus paper.' The rest of us looked scornful and assured her that whatever else the word might mean it could have no possible bearing on urine. The sluices and the Path. Lab. were the place for urine. There was no room for anything so sordid in the Matron's office. We left the problem of 'assiduity' unsolved as we had left so many other problems unsolved over the years.

I felt a lot easier in my mind since I heard that the Matron had been as scathing about the others' progress as she had been about mine. It could only mean that I had not been specially picked on for her censure. Though I knew it was unfair to class me with Davies, Weldon and Baker it made me feel less of an impostor and a let-down to the nursing profession.

I could see that the Irish girl was as pleased as I was. She also was not a born nurse. Her career had been thrust upon her as resolutely as mine had been chosen for me. Our mothers, who had done the thrusting and choosing, had done them for much the same reasons: the main one being that nurses got paid from the start with food and washing thrown in – though not all in together as the flavour of the hospital food suggested. Another was the naïve belief that nursing was a lady-like occupation. They were old-fashioned enough to imagine that nurses whiled away their time flitting round being ladies and laying cool hands on fevered brows. They would have been sadly disillusioned could they have seen us not long after we left our sheltered homes laying freezing cold hands on men's bedwarm bottoms. On my visits home I carefully avoided saying anything that might destroy the picture my mother had of nurses. I told her only the things I thought she would want to hear.

Baker gave her bows a self-conscious little twiddle. 'These bloody things are choking me,' she said, tweaking the tape and shifting a thread that was making inroads into her flesh. We each gave our bows a self-conscious little twiddle, stubbed our cigarettes out on the lino and walked with new-found dignity to the wards.

I was on Female Medical, which suited me fine. I was happy to escape Gynae where the sister got a lot of sadistic pleasure out of bullying new nurses. Having a new staff-nurse to bully would have thrown her into a frenzy of delight. Especially when she saw that the staff-nurse was me. Hers was the first ward that I ever worked on and ever since then we had found little joy in each other's company. There were things on both sides that were best forgotten, even if they could never be forgiven.

I was just as happy not to have been put on a Male ward. Walking through a double row of men with my round chubby face cut off from my round chubby body by a length of tape and a pair of bows was all that the wit of the ward would need to set the rest of the men off laughing. The bows were yet too new to command respect. Given a day or two longer to lose their first crispness they may have spared me some of the cruder comments about my bust and my bottom but not while they were still in their infancy.

The sister on Female Medical greeted me kindly but with no enthusiasm. There was nothing personal about this. She was just not the enthusiastic type. She was small and mousy with a soft face and a gentle voice. The overall impression led the unwary to think that her character would be as colourless as her appearance. Those foolish enough to bank on it were soon having to make a fresh assessment. Beneath the surface softness there was a hard core as steely as my mother's burnished fender. She ran her ward with as much ruthless efficiency as did the sister on Gynae.

The only difference between the two women was that whereas the sister on Gynae stormed and bullied her nurses into abject obedience the sister on Female Medical had more subtle ways of wielding power. She could walk down the ward, head modestly lowered and eyes vigilantly searching, and without a word have all the patients smoothing their top sheets and snatching rubbish off their lockers with as much urgency as if she had browbeaten them into doing it. The technique worked as well with the nurses as it did with the patients.

We rushed to obey her command, did at top speed whatever was commanded, and only realized after it was all done that there had been no command to rush to; or certainly not one that made impact on our ears. We were never quite sure how the message was transmitted: all we knew was that we received it loud and clear. And obeyed.

There was only one thing that disturbed the sister's tranquillity. A nurse had discovered her little weakness one Christmas morning while the staff were congregated in the office drinking the annual celebratory cup of coffee. In the world outside the lodge gates coffee was still a beverage mostly favoured by the leisured classes, the nobility who had scaled the heights, important people like visiting medical staff and very senior sisters; but on Christmas day the beans were brought out, ground down, and distributed like Maundy money round the wards as part of the promotion scheme to get the festivities off to a good start. Most of us would have preferred a nice cup of tea but we suffered the coffee because it was Christmas, and we were supposed to be enjoying ourselves.

'Where do you come from, Sister?' the nurse had asked, emboldened by the heady strength of the coffee and made curious by the faint trace of an accent that crept in whenever the sister was even mildly carried away in conversation. To everybody's amazement she choked into her grouts. She laughed until the tears ran down her cheeks while the nurses stood round not knowing where to look. Nobody had seen the sister behave like this before and it took time to adjust to after her usual unruffled calm. But at last, in an effort to be polite, somebody joined in and gave a restrained little titter. Soon everybody was tittering though they didn't know why. At last the sister told them. 'Nether Wallop,' she gasped, and was off again. Asking the sister on Female Medical where she came from soon became part of the Christmas fun. It made even the coffee taste better.

For the first few months after I became a nurse I walked around in a state of shock. Nothing was easy; life was intolerably hard. My feet killed me, my legs ached, and my heart bled. The new life I had been thrown into at the deep end was so different from anything I had known before that it cast me into deepest despair.

Being a staff-nurse for the first time may not have been so hard on my feet or my legs but there was plenty to make my heart bleed and as much for me to despair over. Suddenly finding myself in a situation where I was expected to dictate instead of being dictated to all the time frightened me to death. I was a follower rather than a leader, content to let others with initiative show me the way. This was to be a great drawback to me in my new role. Other staff-nurses as new as I were able to position themselves at vantage points in the ward and project their voices into the farthest corner and beyond to the usual offices. They could order a junior to 'fetch a bedpan and look sharp about it' with so much authority that the junior downed tools at once to go off at the double and come back at a gallop with the required pan. It didn't work like this for me. I could spend ages looking for a junior, beg her pardon for finding her then humbly ask if she would very much mind going for a bedpan for the patient who had been yelling for one for the past ten minutes. The junior would look so much as if she minded that I invariably finished up begging her pardon again and galloping off for the pan myself. This delighted the juniors and they were as quick to take advantage of it as I would have been under such ineffectual rule.

The sister had me in her office about it one day. She was kind but firm. She always was. She gently pointed out to me that one of the greatest benefits to be derived from becoming a senior was the opportunity it gave to push all the least pleasant jobs on to a junior. This, she said, was called delegating responsibility. She told me that being able to delegate responsibility was as big an asset as the proper use of the powers of observation. Done properly, either could turn a staff-nurse into a sister at an amazing speed. She also reminded me that the reason for the juniors being there at all was because they had an insatiable desire to learn, and if I insisted on doing everything for them they would never learn. I knew that everything she said was true, but knowing did not help. The damage was already done. The juniors continued to look meaningfully in my direction when there was something to be done that they didn't want to do and I continued doing it, as they knew I would if they waited long enough.

The same thing happened whenever I used my powers of observation on them. If I caught them eating or drinking behind the kitchen door when the sister wasn't there it was my duty as a disciplinarian to shriek at them, shout at them, threaten to send them to the Matron, and sort out something particularly nasty for them as a penance for their sins. I did none of these things. I was stopped before I started by vivid mental pictures of myself not so long ago, swallowing lumps of cold cod and slices of plum duff behind a kitchen door, praying earnestly that nobody would come and catch me swallowing. The trouble with me, on top of all my other troubles, was that I could always see two sides of everything and lived in a state of confusion about which side I was on. Getting my bows did little to improve my status; all it did was raise my salary from twenty to twenty-five pounds per year and give me more problems than I had had before.

It was inevitable that Davies and I should share some of the problems. We had been brought up with the same set of rules to abide by and were the victims of the same inhibitions. We were both timid when we should have been bold and strictly teetotal when we should have been sharing the Irish girl's bottle and her parties. The Irish girl was famous for her parties. She was throwing them all the time for the flimsiest of reasons. She started off the celebrations with a full bottle and only brought them to a close when the bottle was empty. None of this was enough to turn her into a raving dipsomaniac. There were always too many guests holding out their tooth mugs for a share of the bottle to make the share-out more than a taster.

During the years that Davies and I had slept in the Irish girl's room while we were still probationers we would never let her talk us into being guests at her parties. When we scented one in the offing, we insisted that she went off with her bottle and drank it somewhere else. Being brought up strictly teetotal we were only too aware of the dangers that befell those who had not signed the pledge and the Irish girl had definitely not signed the pledge. She gave her last party at the hospital soon after she had passed her Finals, not only to mark the occasion but to soften the blow of reminding us that she would soon be leaving.

One morning before we had become staff-nurses we were standing in the library looking gloomily into our empty purses and wondering where the next penny was coming from when the Irish girl got a letter telling us she had won an enormous fortune in the sweepstake. Since the letter contained neither ready cash nor even a small postal order we were still broke and wondering where our next penny was coming from long after the winner had partially recovered from the shock of winning. She never properly recovered. The thought of all that money lying around and her still penniless put her off her food and kept her awake at night, but being twenty-one now she had got her hands on it and was off to America to spend some of it.

At first Davies and I turned down the invitation to the party as we had turned down all previous ones. But, as it was after all a very special occasion and not likely to become a habit, and after the Irish girl had promised to buy us a bottle of lemonade if we would stretch a point and go, we stretched a point and went.

The party was not a success. We sat on the floor in somebody else's bedroom, afraid to turn on the light in case Mary was creeping about. Mary was the sister whose word was law in the home. Only to her face was she called anything but Mary. She did her duty as home-sister with such enthusiasm that nothing but the most infinitesimal escaped her. Though we were of age and entitled to the vote she still insisted on treating us like children in care. We were in for serious trouble if she caught us anywhere but in our own rooms after ten o'clock at night, and far greater trouble if she caught us drinking lemonade in any room at whatever hour. Telling her we were having a party would pour no oil on her troubled waters. Parties were permitted only on Christmas night as a final fling to see us through until the next Christmas night. It would have taken more than a migration to America to persuade Mary to unbend the unbendable rules.

Sitting in the dark may have kept the home-sister at bay but it did nothing to make the convivialities more convivial. The lemonade drinkers quickly segregated themselves from the others and were the first to slake their thirst and abandon the bottle. Thereafter they sat in cold silence on the cold lino while the opposing side sang songs about a woman called Nellie Dean and several green bottles. The silent disapproval soon seeped across the room and the party broke up shortly after it started.

The Irish girl was very bitter about the way things had turned out. She tackled Davies and me about it next morning at breakfast.

'Fine bloody friends you are, I must say,' she said. 'Ruined everything so you did, what with your don't drink this and don't drink that. I wish a thousand times I had never invited you.' We apologized for ruining everything and promised it wouldn't happen again. Then we remembered that because she was leaving it wouldn't happen again anyway and we became a little sad and down in the dumps.

For nearly four years we had smoked each other's cigarettes, borrowed each other's stockings when ours were past darning, laughed, talked, and sometimes cried together. The thought of her leaving suddenly became a minor tragedy; and maybe not so minor at that. We were a close community, drawn closer by a chronic shortage of money and not enough time to join outside communities. The Irish girl had contributed greatly to our happiness, though none of us had appreciated her properly while she had been there. It was only after she went that we realized she was a model of every Irish girl we were to work with over the years: kind, generous and nice to know, and only very occasionally like the Irish jokes that later were to enliven the comedy shows and have audiences falling about in their seats.

'We are going to miss her,' sighed Baker the day before she finally left. We were standing at the uncurtained window in the library. From there we could see the railway bank that had so often provided us with an alternative route into the nurses' home when saying goodnight to boyfriends took longer than it should and we were afraid to face the lodgemen and their menacing pens dipped in ink. Looking down I could almost feel the wet mud caking my knickers as I slithered down a rut after the current boyfriend had given me the push needed to start me on the downward path. But those halcyon days were over. Gone with our butterfly caps and Kirby grips. We were staff-nurses now and the only proper way in for staff-nurses – with examples to set to the juniors – was through the main gates, into the booking-in book, up the drive and through the front door. It was all very respectable and extremely boring.

'We shall certainly miss her swearing,' said Weldon wistfully. 'She is one of the best swearers I've ever heard.' We stood in silence for a moment paying homage to the richness of the Irish girl's language.

'And her a Roman Catholic, is it,' said Davies, breaking the silence and getting a dig in at the Papism that had marred what was otherwise a perfect under- standing between her and the Irish girl. She and Weldon had come in through the front door from the start, Weldon because it was part of her natural good- ness which made her an outstanding friend as well as an outstanding nurse, and Davies because her religious background had remained very much in the fore- ground even though she had stopped going to chapel regularly. They had both disapproved of me for doing such things and were greatly relieved when I passed my Finals and had to give it all up to become respectable.

'I don't care if she is a bloody Roman Catholic, I still say we'll miss her,' said Baker stoutly, and meant it. Though a strict Baptist herself, she knew more ways of getting in late than were dreamed of by Mary and the lodgemen.

None of us were smoking. We had given it up to pool our resources to buy the Irish girl a lighter as a farewell gift. The pool was exceedingly small and the lighter an inferior thing that would have lost its usefulness long before it reached the shores of America. But the Irish girl was touched by the thought, knowing from experience the sacrifices that had been made to buy it for her. She swore that she would cherish it forever, even after she had gone back to lighting her fags with matches.

We saw her off at the station and then walked slowly back, moping a little and talking about her in hushed tones, but by the time her boat had steamed out of the Solent she was pushed to the backs of our minds to make room for other things that were clamouring for attention.

For perhaps longer than we knew there had been rumours circulating about a man called Adolf Hitler. From the things we heard we gathered that he was some sort of German house-painter who had joined the army and worked his way up. The rumours had it that he had worked his way up so high that he was now becoming a force that threatened the world unless something was done to stop him. The thing that mystified us most about it all was how somebody who had so recently been a nobody could cause such a turmoil. To help clear up some of the mystery we started paying more attention to the news bulletins on the wireless and even borrowed newspapers off the patients to read in bed, but we were still little the wiser the night Baker startled us by putting into words the vague fears we were beginning to have.

'What do you think will happen to us when the war breaks out?' she said suddenly while we were eating our supper in the mess-room.

Chapter Two

BECAUSE THE QUESTION had been asked while we were wading through plates of mutton stew it was as hard to digest as the stew would be. However diligently we had followed the political leaders in the papers and however firmly we had rejected the Palm Court orchestras in favour of the news bulletins, we were still not prepared for questions like that. The fact that Baker had said 'when' instead of 'if' made war more of a possibility than a rumoured probability. War was something we would have to study, just as we had studied the nervous system, the circulatory system, and all the other systems while we were doing our training. None of them had come easy to us. The reproductive system was the hardest to grasp. We had started off knowing less about that than we knew about the other systems. Blood and nerves our mothers could steel themselves to mention but reproduction was a closed book, kept carefully hidden from our inquiring eyes. If some of us had dared to open the book in a furtive sort of way at the back of the school bus or during choir practice one evening, what we learnt had confused rather than enlightened us.

'Maybe there won't be a war,' said Weldon hopefully. She had reason for hoping. As well as the trousseau and bottom drawer she was frittering away her salary on, there were the lace curtains to hem for the little house Harry was buying with the two hundred pounds he had managed to save since he bought the engagement ring. War could bring nothing but harm to their plans for the future.

Harry had been mine until I foolishly let him slip through my fingers while I was enjoying a brief but interesting affair with his brother. I had often repented my own folly but I never grudged Weldon her vacant possession of the property I had so wantonly neglected. From the first time I took her with me to his house for tea it had been obvious to everybody that they were made for each other. So beautifully had their voices blended together in an aria from *Madam Butterfly* there were only two or three dry eyes in the room. My voice could never have harmonized with Harry's as Weldon's did. When the time came for her to give him the comfort he needed to assuage the pain I caused him I was quite resigned, and willingly added my sixpence to all the other sixpences that Baker was collecting to buy their engagement present.

Harry was a white-collar worker, earning something in the region of three pounds a week, so with a lot of careful budgeting and sitting up late at night checking the grocery bills Weldon could look forward to a comfortable married life with a home of her own, a baby or two and maybe even a woman in to do the rough. Or thought she could until Baker started asking the question that made her think again.

The answer to the question was as vital to Baker as it was to Weldon. She also was wearing an engagement ring whenever she was off duty long enough to take it out of its little velvet-lined box and put it on. The ring had been given to her by Dr Collins, a dashing young houseman who had seen, heard and been captivated by her when she was still only halfway through her training. It was a foregone conclusion that the wedding ring, the orange blossom and a full choral service would follow close upon her passing her Finals.

Those were the days when a nurse had to have a very good reason for giving up nursing before the letters S.R.N. were appended to her name, if she had started out with any intention of having the letters appended. Marriage was seldom thought to be a good enough reason for abandoning her training somewhere in the middle. But Baker had passed her Finals and had earned the right to put S.R.N. after her name. Until Herr Hitler started shopping round in Austria for *lebensraum* Baker had felt perfectly at liberty to shop around for her wedding dress. We felt sorry for Austria but we felt just as sorry for Baker. Having to re-think your future because a man you knew next to nothing about was threatening a country you knew even less about struck us as being very unfair. It had already begun to look as if the bottom drawer that had been worked on so painfully would have to stay a bottom drawer for ever instead of each garment being lovingly removed, tenderly wrapped in tissue and packed away in a brand-new honeymoon suitcase, ready to set Dr Collins alight with the lacy nightdresses and the feather-stitched petticoats, all done at the expense of much finger-pricking blasphemy. Sewing had never come easy to Baker. It didn't come easy to any of us. Bodging up holes in our black woollen stockings with whatever thread was handy had been the nearest most of us got to sewing a fine seam. Learning how to be a nurse took up too much time to leave us with any for learning other skills.

Weldon mashed up a black and soggy banana that a patient had given her to throw into the pig bin and shared it out between us. We stirred it into our rice pudding, hoping thereby to add a little flavour to the watery half-cooked mixture that lapped the edge of our plate. Without the banana the pudding would have tasted of nothing as most of the food we got in the mess-room did. With the banana it at least tasted of something but it looked terrible.

After we had scooped up the last mouthful and been told by the maids that there was no more left, Davies wiped her mouth on the corner of her apron and looked round at us. Then she said something that churned our stomach as much as the stew and Baker's question had.

'When Archibald came to see me on my day off last week he said he was almost certain there was going to be a war.' She sat back in her chair and gave us time to let the words sink in. We didn't need much time. Archibald was the aristocratic young man she had met while she was nursing his aristocratic old aunt in one of our side-wards. Because of the undoubted blueness of the blood that coursed through his veins the mere mention of his name added weight to the words and made them sink faster. He was, we knew, something terribly important somewhere terribly important in London and we were prepared to believe that if he was almost certain there was going to be a war there most probably would be. If he didn't know what was going on behind the scenes we felt that nobody did.

'He says,' went on Davies, 'if somebody doesn't soon do something to stop that man Hitler he'll go rampaging through everywhere like a steamroller. He says that the only thing that will stop him is for some-body to start standing up to him.' We had a lot on our minds when we went to bed that night.

I stayed awake longer than I had stayed awake since the night before I sat my Finals. Though I had no bottom drawer and no engagement ring to complicate things for me I was as troubled as the others were at the prospect of war. Whenever we had ninepence to spare and an evening off we went to the pictures in the town. We sat through films about the First World War and other wars stretching back through the ages. We sobbed with sobbing sweethearts, wept with weeping wives and rejoiced with returning heroes. It all looked very romantic on the screen but thought of in terms of Baker and Dr Collins, Weldon and Harry, and Davies and her Archibald it lost a lot of its romance. The more I thought about it the less I liked it. Though the films we saw might not have attained the gory reality of techni-color they were graphic enough to give us a vivid picture of what war could be like – fine for glamorous film stars but no good at all for real live (or dead) heroes. I could already see the peace of Female Medical and the strife of Gynae being turned into the horror of wards full of wounded men. I could feel some of the confusion that was lying ahead of us already beginning to close in on me. Suddenly, from a slightly comical little man, with his small moustache, his loud voice and striding jackboots the dream of newspaper cartoonists, Hitler had become real and I was not happy with the sudden reality.

The women on Female Medical were not happy either. They talked of nothing but war. Most of them had sons old enough or husbands young enough to be just the right material for reinforcing the Forces. They all knew this and could envisage the day when their men would be taken from them and used as a brake to check a dictatorship of Nazis on the march through Europe, heels clicking and arm raised in salute to their Leader. Europe was abroad and abroad was a long way away. It was full of foreigners who spoke a funny language and ate peculiar food.

'My father told me,' said one of the women, 'that when he was in France in the last war them Froggies ate snails.' Everybody shuddered at the thought.

'And,' said another, 'I know for a fact they ate horse-meat in Wipers.' More shudders. Froggies eating snails was bad enough but horsemeat in Wipers sounded even more awful.

'What I say is,' said the women, 'let them as wants war go and do the fighting. Why should our men go to foreign parts to die, when they can die just as easy in the pits at home?'

They became even more aggressively British when a German doctor came to work at the hospital. He was a good doctor despite the strange ideas he had about feeding babies. He had strange ideas about a lot of things.

'Throw away the patent foods,' he had said the first time he set foot in the nursery. 'I do not permit such rubbish for babies.' The accent he said it in had to be carefully translated into workable English and even then it was easy enough to get the occasional word wrong. Luckily for us and the patients the word was never one that could become a matter of life and death.

We didn't quite throw away the baby foods. We hid them at the back of a cupboard where the doctor couldn't see them, just in case the babies didn't care much for the substitutes we were offering them. But they did. They swigged their Ovaltine, slurped their Horlicks, guzzled their cocoa and thrived on the new and varied diet. If one of them showed a preference for a drop of warm tea we put the kettle on and made a potful. We never tried them with Guinness but if we had they would no doubt have knocked it back with equal enjoyment.

The doctor had another idea that was just as revolutionary as feeding the babies with whatever was at hand. He firmly believed that given the right treatment it was no longer necessary for new mothers to lie down and die with puerperal fever as they were doing all the time on the Gynae ward. He gave them drugs we had never heard of before and sent them home alive and well instead of to the mortuary or the local lunatic asylum. Until he arrived with his drugs we had nursed puerperal fever according to the textbooks. We tepid sponged, took temperatures, forced fluid through parched lips and warned the husband that there was little hope; then, having done our duty, we had nothing to reproach ourselves with when the mother died, or seemingly recovered, went home and killed the new little baby in a frenzy of puerperal madness.

But none of this counted with the patients when they

discovered that the new doctor was a German. They refused to accept that anybody from a country with a Hitler in it could be anything but as wicked as Hitler. They voiced their feelings and made their protests.

'I'll have none of them bloody Nazis messing about wi' me,' said one of the men when we told him the German doctor was coming to tap his fluid-filled legs. 'How do we know he's not a spy come to find out things so that Jerry can drop a bomb on us as soon as war breaks out?' We didn't know but neither did we think it at all likely. But it was not a bit of good telling this to patients. Soon they were insisting that it had to be someone without a foreign accent who stuck the cold end of his stethoscope on their swelling bosoms or manly chests. And soon even we were beginning to have doubts about the German doctor.

It was rumoured that the reason he left Germany was because he was a Jew. He told shocking things about something called a pogrom that was happening to Jews. He said their homes were being burnt down and their loved ones dragged off to some sort of fearful-sounding camp. We were reluctant to believe him. Jews, Gentiles, Catholics and Protestants were all the same to us. We only ever got bigoted on Sunday mornings, when the Catholics were allowed to go off to Mass, leaving us C. of E.'s, Welsh Calvinists and strict Baptists behind to do all the dirty work.

'It's not fair,' we muttered angrily to each other in the

sluices. 'Why should they be allowed off to go to Mass while we don't even get time to go off for our bread and dripping?' Mass was a constant bone of contention between us.

But apart from that one small ecclesiastical difference none of us could understand why anybody should concern themselves so much with other people's beliefs or ideals. We would have got on just as well with an avowed heathen as we did with the Plymouth Brethren adherent on Male Medical who wore her black stockings off duty as well as on duty instead of keeping a pair of fawn ones for best like the rest of us did.

When the feelings against the German doctor became so strong that he could no longer ignore them he left. We were sad to see him go. We brought out the patent baby food again and went back to tepid sponging the puerperals and soon it was as if he had never been there at all. Except for one young nurse who would remember him with shame for a long time.

He had stormed into Male Medical one morning, taken out a case sheet, examined it closely then turned to the most junior nurse on the ward simply because she was the only nurse in the ward to turn to. He growled something at her in his strong German accent, she failed to understand what he had growled, begged his pardon, missed the repeat and looked wildly round for a senior to take the burden off her. There wasn't one in sight so the poor little junior did her best to make sense of what the doctor was saying. He became as frustrated as she already was. He strode angrily to the medicine cabinet, took out two glycerine suppositories and waggled them under the nurse's nose. 'Take them to the deaf man,' he bellowed, pointing to his ears to emphasize the man's affliction, 'and insert them at once.' The nurse flashed him a grateful smile and tore off to do as she had been shown to do.

The staff-nurse who walked down the ward a little later was astonished to see the deaf man sitting up in bed with a glycerine suppository wedged firmly in each ear. He grew very angry when she questioned him about it.

'I kept telling the silly bitch she should have stuck them up me arse,' he stormed, while the staff-nurse was digging them out of his ears. 'She wouldn't take no notice. She said the doctor had pointed to his ears when he was telling her what to do, not his backside.' The staff-nurse finished making the necessary adjustments then rushed off to report the junior to the sister. The sister spent a long time explaining precisely where a suppository had to go and the junior narrowly escaped being sent to the Matron.

'Lucky for her,' said Baker after we had finished splitting our sides about it. 'My God, if we'd done anything as daft as that while we were juniors we'd have been at the office like a shot. The bloody juniors get away with murder these days.' We nodded agreement, recalling as we nodded the number of times we'd been sent to the Matron for far less and much more than the crime the junior had committed. We spent a happy hour running down the probationers then went off to bed, our haloes bright and our wings bristling with self-righteousness. For, as Davies so piously said, 'If you give them an inch they'll take a yard.' We all agreed that nobody had given us even half an inch while we were probationers.

Rumours went from strength to strength. Soon the thought of war was making the most unlikely people do the most unlikely things. Baker came off duty one evening bursting with excitement.

'Have you heard about the lady almoner?' she asked us. None of us had, which made Baker very happy. It was never as much fun having a tasty bit of gossip to impart if everybody had heard it.

'She's been raped,' she gasped. We refused to believe it. The lady almoner was a very ladylike woman and as necessary to the patients as the Matron was to us. She was also just as terrifying. The idea of anybody doing anything as awful as raping the lady almoner was as hard for us to take in as it must have been for her. We told Baker we didn't believe it. 'But it's true,' she said. 'One of the men who's been in Male San for a long time went to see her this afternoon because his wife's gone off with his best friend. He wanted the lady almoner to go and get her back for him. He'd been in her office for ages then somebody heard her scream. They rushed in and she told them he'd tried to rape her.' We glared at Baker in disgust.

'But you just said she'd been raped,' we reminded her. 'Now you're saying he only tried to rape her.' We were grievously upset at the way the story was going. We had been led to expect the worst and were having to make do with second best.

'Yes, well,' said Baker, sounding embarrassed. 'I wasn't there, was I?' She was conscious that she had promised more than she could deliver. She rallied. 'But even if it was only a try you have to admit it can't have been easy.' We were willing to admit it. Any man brave enough to touch the hem of the lady almoner's serviceable tweed skirt deserved all he got.

It turned out that he hadn't got anything. The true story was exceedingly dull. We would have preferred Baker's version. It seemed that when somebody had loosened the lady almoner's corsets and given her a dose of brandy she looked up and in a weak voice admitted that she might just possibly have made a mistake. What she had taken for a deliberate attempt on her maidenhood may have been nothing more than an accidental brush across the bosom while the man was leaning over her. She re-busked her corsets, drank another dose of brandy and apologized to the man for having confused his elbow with his ardour. Then she put the blame on Hitler and got down to the task of searching for the man's missing wife. It was all over almost before it started.

'A bit of wishful thinking, if you ask me,' said Weldon when the tale was unfolded. 'Pity, though.' We looked at her. 'What's a pity?' asked Davies. 'Well, it might have worked wonders for her,' said Weldon. We thought about it for a moment then the idea of the lady almoner getting therapeutic treatment from a patient instead of him getting help from her had us in stitches.

Not every story had such a happy ending as that one did.

'I'm worried,' said Weldon one evening while we were taking a stroll through the arboretum. We were on nights and had got up early to enjoy what was left of the spring sunshine. We settled ourselves on a bench and lit our cigarettes. 'What are you worried about?' we asked her. 'I don't really know,' she said. 'There's something funny about the runner on my ward and I can't find out what it is.'

'There something funny about all of them,' said Baker, snorting. 'They're lazy, that's what it is. When we were runners we had to run between two and sometimes three wards and nobody worried about us.' We could all remember such nights. But there were other memories that came back to us. Of days spent riding our bicycles down country lanes when we should have been in bed mustering strength for another night's work. We dwelt on those days for a while then listened again to what was worrying Weldon.

'It's not that she's lazy or anything like that. She never stops working. And that's another thing that worries me. It's just not natural.' We got up from the bench and strolled back to the hospital.

A week went by before Weldon mentioned the runner again. 'Do you remember me telling you about that runner I was worried about?' she said, while we were walking across to the wards one night. We remembered well. We had cause to. Mary had caught us going into the home and jumped on us. She had refused to believe for a long time that we had only gone out after four o'clock to take a short walk round the arboretum. When at last she saw that we were telling the truth she had kept us standing while she warned us of the perils that lurked in the bushes in the arboretum. Mary could always be relied on to turn Paradise into a snake-pit. Weldon continued. 'Well,' she said, sounding even more worried than she had been before. 'The other runner who sleeps in her room told me that when she opened one of her drawers by mistake this morning a whole lot of things fell out.'

'What sort of things?' asked Davies. Weldon said the other runner hadn't told her, she just said they were things that a nurse couldn't possibly afford to buy on her first-year salary. Baker gave a sudden start.

'It must be claustrophobia,' she gasped.

'It's not, it's kleptomania,' I told her.

'It's the same thing,' she said.

'Not at all,' I assured her. Baker gave me a dirty look and advised Weldon not to worry. There could, she said, be a perfectly reasonable explanation for the things in the runner's drawers. A rich aunt, a generous godfather, a doting grandma. It was none of these.

When the runner was arrested for shoplifting, a policeman came to the hospital to find out more about her. Mary took him to her room and together they opened boxes and searched through drawers. They found many things that the runner had stolen while she was brooding unhappily over the pain a war could bring to her family with four boys all at the right age for the Services.

We collected enough to pay the fine but she never came back to thank us for it. She went home and we didn't see her again.

It was soon after that Baker came back from her day off looking a lot less cheerful than she usually did.

'Gran and Grandad are moving soon,' she told us when we asked her what was wrong. She was devoted to her grandparents. They lived in the same street as her father and mother and in the same house they had lived in all their married life.

'But they've always lived there,' we said. 'Why on earth should they suddenly decide to move?' Baker took off her best dress and hung it in the wardrobe. She kicked her shoes across the room and Davies went over and picked them up. Baker thanked her. 'That's what I asked them,' she said. 'Grandad says that when the war breaks out Coventry will be one of the first places it will hit.' We were as doubtful about that as we had been about the lady almoner story. Then Baker went on to tell us more unbelievable things.

'They're sending all the children away as well,' she said. 'There were hundreds of them on the platforms. They had gas masks in cardboard boxes and labels round their necks to tell people who they were and where they were going. Some of them were going all the way to Wales. It was awful. I couldn't bear to look at them. The children were crying, their mothers were crying and you'd have cried as well if you'd been there.' We gathered from the defiant way she said it that she also had cried a little.

When her grandparents moved they took their parrot with them. It had been with them since it was a baby and they couldn't bear to leave it behind. Baker read a letter to us later. It said that the parrot didn't swear like it used to. It only swore when it was happy and it wasn't happy any more. Neither were Baker's gran and grandad. Neither was anybody. The threat of war hung like a great black cloud. It was expected to break out at any minute.

Chapter Three

BUT THERE WASN'T to be a war after all – or so they told us. Mr Chamberlain flew off to Germany, had cosy little chats with Herr Hitler, and came back waving his umbrella about and making optimistic prophecies about peace in our time. Whose time he had in mind he omitted to mention, certainly not his with a few more years still to go, and surely not ours with a lifetime of living ahead of us. But peace. So, while Hitler stomped around, frightening everybody with his stomping, we kept ourselves to ourselves as my mother would have said and refrained from sticking our nose into other people's business. Which made the women on Female Medical very happy, except for the thinking ones who thought that Mr Chamberlain might be wrong.

Because war hadn't broken out as we expected it to, I, and a lot of other people, went back to making plans for the future. One of the first plans I made was to go and ask the Matron for permission to live out.

Living out was one of the rights we earned when we

passed our Finals. It was not a right that the Matron wholeheartedly approved of. Getting her permission to pack our bags and leave the nurses' home was almost as difficult as getting her permission to come and live there in the first place. It made begging for a late pass or supplicating for a sleeping-out pass ridiculously easy by comparison; notwithstanding the fact that having to beg and supplicate kept us awake the night before we did it.

The reason I decided to try my luck at living out was because I was rapidly running short of excuses to give the lodgemen when they glared ferociously at me from beneath bushy eyebrows and insisted on being told why I was creeping in at three minutes past ten on my evenings off when the statutory time was ten. Over the years they had become more and more sceptical about buses that broke down, buses that had not run at all, and buses that unaccountably took wrong turnings somewhere, leaving me to trail back late to the hospital. They exhibited frank disbelief at my touching little stories about helping old ladies across the road or giving first aid to the man who practically dropped dead at my feet. They had heard it all before and, however noble the cause that had delayed me, they were waiting pen dipped in ink to put a black mark against my name for the Matron to see and frown over when she inspected the booking-in book in the morning. It occurred to me that the only way I could escape the lodgemen was to go and live somewhere where there were no lodgemen. After giving it some thought I told the others of my plan while we were in the Kardomah drinking Russian tea one morning.

We had been drinking Russian tea in the Kardomah on and off for a long time. Usually on the beginning of the month while we could still afford it, and off at the end when we couldn't afford anything. With practice we had become less self-conscious about the slice of lemon that was wedged on the side of the glass. We either left it where it was or we removed it and scraped the juice out with a long-handled spoon they gave us, perhaps for that very purpose. Though we had acquired a little taste for the tea we were still not over-fond of it; we drank it rather for effect than pleasure. Davies had taken longer to get used to it than we had. For a long time she refused to believe that the lemon was a substitute for the milk and insisted on adding both. The resultant clots that floated to the top curled her nose and put her off her tea. We eventually managed to educate her into putting in the lemon and leaving out the milk but it took a long time.

For various reasons we had stopped going to the more expensive cafés in the town. I was the first to lose interest in them when the romantic violinist I had once mooned over turned out to be the father of many, each the spitting image of him – without his violin, of course. The others stayed away after it had dawned on them that somebody was having to pay for the string ensemble that fiddled and strummed on the dais. It didn't take much mathematical genius to work out that it was poverty-stricken people like us that were subsidizing its up-keep.

A cup of tea could cost as much as tuppence with the *Blue Danube* thrown in, which mightn't be too bad if somebody else was footing the bill but could make a considerable dent in our salaries if we were meeting the cost. A bun in one of the plushier places was quite out of the question.

There was no ensemble at the Kardomah so, by missing out on the strings, we could occasionally run to a slice of angel cake; its three layers of melt-in-the-mouth lightness, pink and white and gummed together with gooey cream all unbearably tantalizing when we saw it on the counter protected from the dust by a funereal glass dome. The angel cake was well worth sacrificing our musical education for. We were forking up the last crumbs of a slice when I broke the news.

'I am thinking of asking the Matron if I can live out,' I announced, stacking sugar in my tea with nonchalance that fooled nobody. Weldon, Davies and Baker laid down their pastry forks and stared at me.

'What on earth for?' asked Baker, for once forgetting to remind me that sugar was fattening and no wonder I could not get clothes to fit me.

I was not anxious to go into my reasons for wanting

to live out. None of them would have understood. Weldon and Davies never needed to come in late and even Baker had mended her ways after she got engaged to Dr Collins. Not so much through virtue but because being a doctor he could open doors that were closed to us.

Davies saved me the trouble of having to think up reasons. 'She'll never let you,' she said sounding extremely opposed to the idea.

'She'll have to,' I told her. 'We're allowed to live out when we've passed our Finals and there's not a thing she can do about it.' We all knew there was plenty she could do about it if she wanted to – like saying 'No' for example.

'Where are you thinking of living?' asked Weldon, licking buttercream off her fingers. This was another question I could have wished they hadn't asked. I'd given no thought to where I was going to live. I'd given no thought to the seamier side of living out. I started giving it some thought.

'Oh, I'll find somewhere, I expect,' I said, already beginning to wonder where.

'But where?' pressed Weldon. 'The Matron will want to know where you're going to live before she'll let you go.' I knew she was right. Despite her aloofness the Matron had our welfare very much at heart. I thought fast for an answer that would satisfy both her and my inquisitors.

'We've got a patient on Female Medical who says she takes in lodgers,' I said. 'I could ask her if she'll take me in.'

'What's she like?' asked Davies, who also had my welfare at heart. 'Is she clean and all that?' For her cleanliness had the edge on godliness if the choice were to be made.

'Well,' I said thoughtfully, 'she has a good wash down when we give her a bowl in the morning and she always uses two flannels.' Using two flannels, one for either end of the anatomy, put a patient on a higher social scale from those who used the same flannel for top and bottom. Davies seemed satisfied with the character reference I gave my future landlady and I hoped the inquisition was over. It wasn't.

'Where does she live?' Baker wanted to know. I hadn't the least idea. I hadn't examined her case sheet long enough to find out. I confessed as much.

'Suppose she lives miles away from the hospital and you have to pay for a bus to get there and back,' said Davies, making it sound as if I was in the market for the outright purchase of a bus. Davies could be very discouraging sometimes. She had an infuriating habit of casting shadows when she should have been throwing light.

'I shall just have to give up smoking,' I said in an attempt to quell their fears about my financial situation. They gave sardonic laughs.

'Well, all right then,' I said desperately, 'we don't know where the woman lives yet, do we? She might only live a stone's throw from the hospital: then I can walk there and back.'

'Fat chance,' said Davies.

We went carefully over the bill, checking for possible overcharging, then we shared a shilling equally between us and ran to catch the bus back to the hospital. We left no tip on the saucer. We never did. We had decided long ago that nobody tipped us for the things we did for them, and we did as much – even more – than the waitresses did for us.

That night, while we were sitting on Baker's bed talking about Dr Collins, Harry and Archibald, I managed to change the subject and bring the others up to date with my living-out plans.

'I talked to the woman who takes in lodgers this afternoon while I was giving her an enema and she says it's quite all right. I can go whenever I like.' Baker glared at me in disgust.

'Why on earth were you giving her an enema?' she asked furiously. 'Enemas are things that are supposed to be delegated to juniors, aren't they?' I hastily explained that the only place we could have a little chat with a patient on my ward was behind a screen where the sister couldn't see us. She had strict rules about us not talking to the patients. She often reminded us that they were there to be nursed not to be talked to. Except for saying 'Is it yes?' which was her polite way of asking if the bowels had been opened that day the sister rarely exchanged a word with a patient. But she nursed them devotedly.

Davies laid aside her sewing for the moment and gave her full attention to me and the woman who took in lodgers.

'I still think you ought to find out a bit more about her before you go to lodge with her,' she said. 'Supposing she's awful when you get there. You can't always tell when they're lying in bed.' As usual Davies was right. Once they were in their winceyette and settled back on the pillows they took on a new look; often it was a look of martyrdom coupled with a gratified awareness of their sudden importance, unless of course they were brought in too ill to be aware of anything.

The new look, together with the mass-produced sameness of the winceyette, resulted in greater social equality than Socialism would ever achieve.

Persuaded by Davies and egged on by the others, I waited until the woman on Female Medical had been home for a day or two then I went to see her. Davies had warned me not to say anything to the woman about the visit in case she made special preparations for it – like tidying up the place or going over it with a quick flick of a duster.

The woman who opened the door to my knocking

looked nothing at all like the woman I'd given the enema to. She had on a torn pinny over a grubby dress and her hair was a mass of Dinky curlers. The smell that came out of the small dark passage was worse than the smell in the mess-room if there had been cabbage for dinner recently. I stood back a few inches to avoid the blast. There must have been cabbage on the menu for a long time.

The woman didn't recognize me at first. She was as used to seeing me in my starch and stripes as I was to seeing her in her nightdress. It was a few minutes before I was able to establish my identity.

'Well, who'd a' thought o' seeing you?' she said at last, delightedly. 'Come in, do. I was just going to put the kettle on and make meself a cup o' tea.' We felt our way through the passage and into the kitchen. She poked the fire and set a blackened kettle on the sulky coals. Then she looked round for somewhere for me to sit. There was nowhere. Every inch of sitting space in the room was taken up by cats. There were cats on the horsehair sofa, cats lolling languorously on the matching chairs and a cat on each of the two foot-stools. There were others lying peacefully on the table.

'Shoo,' said the woman, waving her hand vaguely round the room. Not a cat stirred. The woman tried again, this time using threats.

'Naughty pussies,' she said sternly. 'Mother's going to get very angry with pussies if pussies don't get up and let the lady sit down.' When mother's threatened anger failed to move the cats she turned to me with a merry laugh.

'Bless their dear little hearts,' she said fondly. 'Who could get mad with the little darlings?' I could, I thought, easily. But I was no cat lover. On the farm where I had spent my childhood the sole purpose of keeping cats was to stop the barn being overrun by mice and in the nurses' home Mary would have had a fit if anything so alien as a cat had put its nose round the door. Not to mention Nellie the housemaid. She couldn't abide cats at any price, she told us once. Not since the day her sister was frit to death by one and her expecting at the time. When the baby was born, Nellie said, it was as hairy as a kitten. Luckily it had grown out of it since and become a soldier. But Nellie would never forget it, not if she lived to be hundred. Nellie told us a lot of stories like that, and though we never doubted them for one moment they stretched our imaginations to the limit sometimes.

When the kettle started spitting and sizzling on the fire the woman made the tea. She let it brew for ten minutes while we talked then she poured it through the rubber spout of a grimy teapot into two cracked cups. She spooned a quantity of sweetened condensed milk from a sticky tin into the tea, gave the spoon a good lick then vigorously stirred the tea with the well-licked spoon. She seemed quite upset when I apologized and said I didn't drink tea, especially after all the trouble she'd been to to make it for me.

I stood around for a while longer, getting buffeted around by two cats and a large dog that had come into play with the resident cats, and then I said I had better be going and I would let the woman know as soon as I got the Matron's permission to live out. I said it in a way that could but sow seeds of doubt about my being able to get the necessary permission. The woman led me out through the cabbage-scented hall and I never went back there again.

The others were waiting for me agog for news. I told them about the curlers, the cabbage, the cats and the tinned milk and they each in turn and in their separate ways said I told you so. After that I gave up the whole idea of going to live out and concentrated instead on thinking up fresh excuses to give to the lodgemen when I came in late.

The next to take advantage of Mr Chamberlain's 'peace in our time' was Baker. Her plans, though made in haste, were never repented. She told us about them one night while we were eating our midnight meal.

Chapter Four

WE WERE THROUGH the mince and well on into the rice pudding when Baker shocked us by telling us she was getting married the following morning. At first we thought she was joking. She had to be joking. There was no possible way that she could be single tonight and married tomorrow and us knowing nothing about it until that moment. Then we looked at her and saw that her eyes were shining. We realized she wasn't joking, she was in deadly earnest.

'But why?' we asked. 'Why so suddenly? And why haven't you said anything about it before?' The vision we'd had of her with veil and orange blossom, walking sedately down the aisle, began to fade.

Baker put down her spoon. The rice pudding was less fluid than it usually was. Instead, it was all stodge and starch. I liked it better that way, but Davies liked it runny. Baker preferred it midway between stodge and liquid. 'It's because of the war,' she said. 'There's going to be a war, in spite of everything that old woman Chamberlain says. And when it comes it'll come suddenly and there will probably be no time for things like white weddings, so we're going to do it now, before it's too late.' After she had finished talking we knew that she was indeed going to be married tomorrow, or even today if it was already past midnight. None of our watches were in working order and there was no clock in the mess-room. Most of our timing was done by instinct. It seldom let us down. Through practice we were able to assess within a single heartbeat the rate of a pulse, simply by gazing down at our stopped watches. Having them repaired cost money, and money was something we had never enough of.

'You still haven't told us why you haven't told us before,' said Weldon. Telling us before would have given us time to club together and buy her a wedding present. It would also have put a considerable strain on our finances, already strained with buying Weldon an engagement present. But we would have willingly strained everything to its uttermost for Baker.

'I couldn't tell you before,' she said. 'I didn't know myself until yesterday.' The reason she hadn't known was that Dr Collins didn't tell her until he had bought a special licence and got it all fixed up at the register office. Then, when it was all arranged and too late for Baker to argue about, he told her. He knew he was safe. He knew that anything he did would meet with her approval, even if it meant abandoning the full choral service and the peal of bells we had been anticipating so eagerly.

We sat silent for a moment, stunned by the romance that had crept into our midnight meal. Then Weldon brought us back to earth.

'But surely you'll have to leave when the Matron knows?' she said. 'She'll never let you stay on once you're married.' Being a wife as well as a nurse was not yet approved of by hospital training schools. The day of a nurse being wife and mother had still to dawn. We little knew then how close the dawn was. Baker went pale.

'She mustn't know,' she said anxiously. 'You must swear not to breathe a word to anybody, then she'll never find out.' None of us needed to swear. We had been Baker's friends too long to have to do anything as dramatic as that. We each swore a solemn and binding oath.

There were more shocks in store for us the next morning when we came off duty. Baker bundled us into the library and shut the door, standing guard against it in case Mary or Nellie, who spied for her, was anywhere within earshot. Nellie was one of the domestics in the home. She was Mary's right-hand woman. And her faithful informant.

'I want you to come with me to the register office and be witnesses,' Baker said. 'There need only be two, but you might as well all come. There won't be anybody else there, it was too sudden to tell them at home.' The thought of being witnesses instead of going to bed was thrilling enough to stop us yawning, though not thrilling enough to quell our fears.

'What if Mary catches us going out?' we inquired anxiously. 'She'll go mad if she sees us going out of the home when we ought to be in bed.' Though we had become staff-nurses we still tried to avoid running the risk of sending Mary mad. Her madness could be an awesome sight.

'You'll do as you always do,' hissed Baker, with one eye on the door. 'You'll wait until she's round stripping the day nurses' beds, then you'll sneak out through the back entrance, hide behind a car or something going up the drive and meet me outside the gates at ten o'clock.' She made it sound easy. And so it was for her. She was off that night and didn't have to worry about colliding with Mary on the doorstep. Nor did she have to think up ways of dodging the lodgeman.

'How shall we dodge the lodgeman?' we asked feebly. Baker gave us a withering look. It was a look we deserved. For, as she said, if we didn't know after all these years how to get out without the lodgeman seeing us it was a bad job. And especially for something as important as her wedding. We apologized for our inadequacies. We had come off duty after a busy night. The smallest molehill loomed as large as a mountain.

We got out of the home and up the drive without a voice of thunder halting us or a heavy hand arresting us in our progress. We were less fortunate when we reached the lodge. The man in it was one of the more alert of our warders. He knocked on his window, threw it open, looked us up on his list and asked furiously why we was going out at that time of a morning when we knew as well as he did that we were on nights and supposed to be in bed. With the help of a few cigarettes that we raked up between us we managed to get him on our side and he let us through the gates. Baker was waiting for us outside.

She looked extremely pretty. She was wearing her everyday clothes, except for a pair of stockings with no holes in them, and the pink straw hat trimmed with daisies she had worn for her sister's wedding. Her hair was fluffed out at the sides in a most becoming way. She told us shyly that she was wearing one or two oddments from her bottom drawer under her dress and showed us a bit of lace to prove it. This delighted a passing motorist and he honked the horn of his Austin Seven in masculine appreciation of the leg show.

The register office was in a dreary part of the town. The exterior was in keeping with the environment. The interior was even more depressing.

We climbed up a narrow staircase and followed an arrow marked 'Marriages'. There was also an arrow marked 'Births' and another marked 'Deaths'.

The 'Marriages' arrow pointed directly into a dingy waiting-room where there were several people standing about or sitting down, all looking very uncomfortable. At a quick glance we could quite easily have landed at the terminal point of the 'Deaths' arrow.

We were just about to turn round and clarify our position when we noticed a girl in a far corner of the room. She was unmistakably a bride. She wore a full-length satin gown with a tulle train and an orange-blossomed coronet. With no pageboys or bridesmaids to take responsibility for the train it trailed dejectedly on the dusty floor. A large bouquet of red roses sat by its side.

The groom looked very young. He seemed hot and uncomfortable in his very new soldier uniform. It was obvious that he, like Dr Collins, had brought things forward before Hitler started pushing them too far back.

The bride's mother had the numbed look of a woman still trying to recover from the shock of having to renounce the pomp and ceremony of St Michael's and All Angels with a buffet do in the hall to follow. She dabbed at her eyes and fiddled with the carnation in her buttonhole and tried to dissociate herself from the people around her. She was definitely above them.

We had been sitting there for a few minutes when Dr Collins came in. His eyes were deep with tiredness. He had been up most of the night trying to avert yet another tragedy on Gynae. He had failed to avert it. He sat beside Baker and they held hands while we waited.

When the call came for us to go through the door marked 'No Smoking' we all put out our cigarettes and trooped into the room. It was very small. It was also dingy, dirty, flyblown and bare. The few fixtures and fittings consisted of six chairs arranged in two sets of three, a desk, and a gaunt-looking man who sat on a seventh chair behind the desk. From his appearance we could see that he divided his time fairly between the three arrows. He wore a shiny black suit, a black tie frayed at the edges, a pair of bright canary-coloured socks and co-respondent shoes in two shades of cream. Separately, each item might have been passable, but together they screamed their incompatibility.

The man instructed Davies, Weldon and me to disperse ourselves among the chairs on the visitors' side while he arranged Baker and Dr Collins before him at the desk, the better to see them while he was marrying them.

Immediately above the chair I was sitting on there hung a flypaper. It was liberally spattered with the corpses of its victims. So densely populated was it that newcomers had trouble in finding accommodation for themselves. They jostled the dead to get at the treacle that daubed the flypaper. The dead fell on my lap and as fast as I brushed them off more fell. In the end I stopped worrying about them and allowed them to rest in peace.

It took the man several minutes to get us where he wanted us to be and when he had he flicked through some documents on the desk, polished the toes of his shoes on his trouser leg, blew his nose, gazed mournfully at the result then finally composed himself to address Dr Collins. What he said I never heard. At the precise moment that he opened his mouth a sash cord broke and the window fell down with a shattering crash. Davies, Weldon and I leapt from our chairs and looked round in panic. We were absolutely certain that war had broken out the way everybody said it would. The Registrar went on addressing Dr Collins as if nothing unusual had happened. He made it seem as if a sash cord breaking was one of the hazards of getting married, which, considering the state of the register office, could have been possible.

If the incident had done nothing to put the Registrar off his stroke it had destroyed the little confidence that Dr Collins had mustered. He dropped the ring, bent to pick it up, dropped it again and looked beseechingly at Baker to rescue him from his predicament. With a face sweet with love she picked up the ring and prompted him when he forgot his lines. And when it was her turn she went through it all without once faltering. When it was over her eyes were alight with happiness beneath the pink straw hat.

Dr Collins bought the wedding breakfast at a shop near the register office. He dashed in and came out with a bag of currant buns, one for each of us. He apologized for not having enough money to buy a bottle of lemonade but we said that it would be quite all right, we would wash the buns down with water. He ate his while he was standing there, then he gave Baker a gentle kiss on the cheek and rushed to get back to the hospital before too many people realized he had ever been away from it. We returned at a more leisurely pace. We got in safely. The lodgeman raised his eyebrows but since he had one of our cigarettes dangling from his mouth there was nothing he could do about it except glare. Mary was busily occupied catching out a sinner in some other part of the home.

Because it was Baker's wedding day we accepted her invitation to go to her room to eat the wedding breakfast instead of going straight to bed. We ate the buns and drank water from her toothmug. We talked about the ceremony and said how lovely it had all been; we told Baker she had looked beautiful in the pink straw hat with daisies on it, then we waited for someone to ask the question we were all dying to ask. It was Weldon who at last plucked up courage.

'What are you doing about a honeymoon?' she mumbled through her bun. We averted our eyes from Baker. Honeymoons were sex, and sex was something we didn't talk about openly to each other. Though we were brought face to face with it in its various forms on the wards it was still something we fought shy of mentioning freely. Only Pickford had ever brought it into general conversation and none of us was a Pickford.

Baker went scarlet and almost choked over the bite of bun she had in her mouth. We had to wait a long time before she could get it down and come up with an answer.

'I'm not quite sure,' she said at last. 'He did suggest that I popped over to the doctors' quarters later on. When there was nobody about, of course.' She took another gulp of water and passed round the toothmug. We each took a gulp of water. Now that the sexual hurdle was safely over there was less tension in the air.

'But how can you pop over there?' asked Weldon, aghast. 'It's out of bounds except on Christmas night.' Even on Christmas night the licensing hours were short and subject to certain conditions. There was a large plaque on the door of the doctors' quarters. On it was written 'Nurses not allowed in the doctors' quarters except on Christmas night, and then only in uniform and not later than ten p.m.' The wearing of the uniform was of vital importance. It ensured that the doctors wouldn't have their passions unbridled by the sight of a nurse minus her starched front.

The 'ten p.m.' was an extra deterrent. Mary and the Matron had lived long enough and seen enough of the world to know only too well the awful things that could happen to a girl once the stroke of ten died down. They were determined to save us from ourselves, and from all things pleasurable. We thought of Baker popping over to the doctors' quarters and trembled. I had a sudden inspiration.

'Why can't he pop over here instead?' I asked. 'He knows all the ways into the home and if he heard Mary or the night sister on the warpath while he was here he could jump out of the window and run back.' There were enough sandbags stacked up outside the window to provide a launching pad for an enterprising and lithe young man like Dr Collins. Baker considered the idea.

'But how am I going to let him know?' she asked, looking worried. 'He's expecting me to pop over there and he'll wonder where I am if I don't.' We promised her faithfully that by hook or by crook we'd get the message across to him, then we scraped up the bun crumbs, ate them and stumbled wearily to bed, leaving Baker to get used to the idea of being Mrs Dr Collins.

That evening we got up feeling miserable. Long before midnight we were wishing it was morning and by morning we were wishing we could go to bed for a week.

Before we finally went to bed we decided to visit Baker to find out how she'd slept. Put delicately like that the question would cause her no embarrassment.

If she didn't want to tell us anything she didn't have to, but if she did bring herself to make a few disclosures it might make interesting listening. We tapped very gently on her door.

She looked very angry when we walked in. There was nothing of the blushing bride about her.

'You forgot!' she stormed furiously.

'Forgot what?' we asked.

'You forgot about telling him to pop over here.' We looked at each other. It was true. We were so bad-tempered when Nellie called us for duty that we hadn't given a thought to Baker's honeymoon. She went on storming for a long time before she forgave us. When she did we made her promise that she would put a good word in for us with Dr Collins when he threatened to kill us the next time he saw us.

Later that morning the Matron sent for Baker. She told us about it later.

'She knew,' she said. 'She knew all about me being married.' We looked at each other, wondering which one of us had turned traitor. None of us had. When we thought about it afterwards we could only conclude that Nellie had seen Baker going out in her best fawn stockings and the pink straw hat with daisies on it and had managed to add two and two together. Though there were things that Nellie wasn't too bright about, even she knew that nurses didn't go out in their best stockings in the morning unless there was something very special happening. And the daisy-trimmed hat told its own story. Our usual headgear was a navy blue beret, with maybe a red one for best.

But the most amazing thing to transpire out of Baker's visit to the Matron was that the Matron hadn't been too out of her mind with anger at the marriage. Naturally she had to do her duty and tell Baker off. She couldn't have her nurses running off to get married without taking some stand against it. But when she had finished taking the stand she had a long talk with Baker.

She said that though she didn't approve of nurses getting married times were changing, and she would obviously have to change with them. But not too much, she hoped. She said that Baker would have to go and live out, and take Dr Collins to live out with her. She also suggested that it might be a good idea if they postponed the honeymoon until a more suitable venue was found for it. Baker said that as well as all the other things she knew, she seemed to know that there had been no to-ing and fro-ing from the doctors' quarters. She seemed quite pleased about this, Baker said. We were pleased that the Matron was pleased. It made us feel less guilty about not delivering the message to Dr Collins.

'It must be something to do with the war,' said Weldon. 'They must be realizing they'll need all the nurses they can get when the war breaks out.'

'Like they did in the Crimean war,' said Davies. I reminded her that there had been wars since the Crimean and told her all I knew about Edith Cavell. I knew very little, but luckily Davies knew even less.

When Harry's mother heard that Baker was married and wanted somewhere to live she cleaned out her spare bedroom and offered it to her. The spare room was the one her other son would have been sleeping in if he hadn't already given his life for a Cause that none of us had known much about. In those days Spain was as distant as Austria.

Having a pair of newly-weds sleeping in the next room to him must have kindled a flame in Harry. It wasn't long before Weldon was inviting us to a wedding that would take place in the not too distant future. Harry had a less impulsive nature than Dr Collins, and the date for the wedding was distant enough to give us time to collect for the set of EPNS fruit spoons. To go with the fish knives and forks we'd given them when they got engaged.

I bought a pair of white gloves and some new stockings to wear to the church, and freshened up my old coat with a damp rag. I could have saved myself the trouble and expense. On the day of the wedding I was living it up in sick bay with measles. I lent Davies the gloves and stockings. She told me all about it after I got out of sick bay. She said that Weldon looked lovely walking up the aisle in the shimmering dress her mother had worn at her wedding. The train was held up by Harry's little sister and several small cousins, and there was a proper reception with a three-tiered cake. Weldon and Harry had sung a duet together then had gone off to Llandudno for a week. It all sounded very nice and I was sad that I hadn't been there to see it for myself.

Chapter Five

THE MEASLES THAT had been threatening all morning finally came to a head while I was laying a linseed poultice on a patient's wheezing chest. I had rushed the poultice from kitchen to bedside between two dinner plates, thereby ensuring that the linseed would keep hot enough to make the patient say 'ooh' and 'aah' when I slapped it on. I was in no mood for sympathizing with her oohs and aahs. I was too busy feeling sorry for myself.

I had got up that morning with a raging headache, two burning eyes and a throat that felt as if it had been rubbed down with wet-and-dry. When I tried explaining to the sister how awful I felt and suggested that it might be better if I went back to bed, or at least stayed off the ward until whatever I was suffering from was diagnosed she dismissed the symptoms as the usual tricks that nurses got up to when they felt like having time off work. She promised me that if I worked hard enough I would forget all about it. While she was making the promise I thought of the time when I was doing my training and a sister had said the same things to Mannering. Mannering had died instead of getting better. I was morbidly certain the same thing was about to happen to me.

The woman I was almost scalding with the red-hot poultice had at last become resigned to having the first layer of delicate skin torn from her chest and had begun talking of other things. The things she was talking about caught and held my attention. Though they were pitched in a lower key than her protests I was more prepared to listen to them.

'What will you do when the war starts?' I heard her ask. The patients had gone back to talking about war when they saw that in spite of Mr Chamberlain's optimism sandbags were still being piled up and air-raid shelters built. Though some of the children had been taken home again when it seemed there would be nothing for them to flee from there was still a feeling that nothing would ever be quite the same as it had been before the crisis year.

'I expect I'll be doing much the same as I'm doing now,' I said drearily, smoothing the wrinkles in her draw sheet and helping her on with her nightdress. I had been smoothing wrinkles in draw sheets for so long that I could see no reason at that moment why I should ever be doing anything different. The throbbing head had something to do with the dreariness.

'Of course you won't,' said the woman, trying frantically to get her head out of the armhole where she had forced it. 'It'll all be different when the war comes.' We rescued the head from the armhole and almost broke an arm pushing it into the vacant space. 'When the war comes there'll be bombs and things, and everybody will be blown up or gassed. There'll be no room in hospital then for bronchitics like me.' She lay back on the pillows, conscious that she had said enough to pay me out for the torture I had put her through. Meticulously I measured the turn-back of the top sheet and fiddled with it until it was the exact width the sister insisted it should be, then I tucked everything in so tightly the woman could hardly breathe. The more easily she was able to breathe the less perfect was the bed-making.

'They wouldn't dare to do things like that,' I said. 'They'd be afraid we'd do the same to them.' The minute I said it I realized that I was turning war into a game played by children. The woman took a comb from her locker and dragged it through her bobbed hair, tousled with being pulled through the armhole. She looked at me pityingly.

'Don't you believe it, duck,' she said. 'Them Jerries is ready for anything we can do to them. It'll be us as won't be ready, you mark my words.' I did an exceedingly poor hospital corner with the ends of her counterpane then checked carefully to make sure that the pillowslip openings were not on the side facing the ward door. The width of the turn-back of the sheet, the precision of the corners of the counterpanes and the positioning of the ends of the pillowslips were important enough to make or mar a ward report. Checking on them took up a lot of the sister's time. 'Openings away from the door, Nurses,' she would cry if she saw so much as a hint of ticking peeping at her when she walked into the ward. Should she have any doubts about the turn-back she measured it carefully with her arm. The required width was the exact distance from her elbow to the tip of her middle finger. A centimetre out could cause it to be done again.

'But suppose they did drop bombs and use gas, they wouldn't be doing it on us,' I assured the woman with the assurance of ignorance. The woman made a slight scoffing sound.

'Don't you believe it,' she said. 'The day is over when them as starts the wars goes and fights them. When this lot starts we'll all be in it.' I refused to believe her. I reminded her that in the films they showed us at the pictures battles were fought on proper battlefields. What about Flanders, I asked, and Wipers, and all the other places that were only names and not even properly pronounced names?

'Well, all right then,' said the woman. 'If you don't believe me, what about them air-raid shelters they're building, and all them gas masks they're giving out? What do you make of that then?' What I made of it astonished me as much as it dismayed her. I sat on the bed and burst into tears.

The woman was as shocked at seeing me crying as we had been at seeing the sister laughing. It was so removed from her concept of how nurses should behave that it was some time before she could make up her mind what to do about it.

'Are you feeling poorly, duck?' she asked at last, giving me a nervous little pat on the back. The kindness of her voice and the nervous little pat did nothing to dry my tears. I threw myself on to the poultice I had just applied and wept bitterly. At first the woman drew herself away. It was as big a sin for a patient to become too familiar with a nurse as it was for a nurse to become too familiar with a patient. Such straying from what was proper could bring bad trouble all round. But suddenly she became a mother and saw in me a woeful girl rather than an impersonal nurse. She enfolded me in her arms and rocked me gently.

The news that there was a nurse in tears behind the screens spread through the ward and down to the sister's office. She hurried down, tore me from the woman's arms and marched me from the ward. She told me to stop being so ridiculous and reminded me that I was a nurse and that for a patient to witness a nurse behaving in such a stupid way could destroy the very fabric of nursing as Miss Nightingale knew it. After she had said a few more things she peered into my face and shrank back in alarm.

'Really, Nurse,' she exploded. 'Why didn't you tell me when you came on duty that you didn't feel well? Didn't it ever occur to you that you might have measles? You may have infected the whole ward. Go across to the home at once and report to sick bay.' I went. Shamefaced and spotty. Having the terrible responsibility laid upon me of infecting the whole ward made my head throb even more.

Mary, who was the custodian of sick nurses as well as healthy ones, refused to believe at first that there was anything wrong with me. After she had first accused me of being a chronic hypochondriac then of using the war scare as an excuse to malinger, she at last noticed the spots. She gave a shriek and demanded to know why the sister hadn't sent me across sooner. It could be seen at a glance, said Mary, that I had measles, and only a fool like the ward sister could have missed it. Now, she said, there was a chance that I might have infected the whole hospital. She flung some sheets and blankets on a bed and I crawled into it. When my aching head was at last resting on a pillow I realized that it took a lot of courage to go off sick. There also had to be spots to back up the claim. Without the spots I would have still been on duty, however ill I felt.

The others were very disappointed in me for only having measles. When Baker saw my red eyes and flushed face at breakfast time she had immediately diagnosed diphtheria. She had taken us step by step through the post-operative treatment of a tracheotomy including all the complications that could arise. Measles was a poor substitute for the drama of an emergency tracheotomy. Once again I had failed to do what was expected of me. I felt very low.

Nevertheless, that evening they came and stood on a box outside sick bay window, which was the nearest Mary would allow them to get to me, and threw a small parcel on to my bed. In the parcel was a canvas tea cosy with a little thatched cottage and some hollyhocks stencilled on it, a few hanks of embroidery wool and a crewel needle. There was also a hastily scribbled note telling me what a hoot I looked in spots.

I whiled away the next ten days stabbing wool through the canvas and imagining the delight on my mother's face when she saw the finished product. She never did see it. The moment the last spot had gone Mary had the tea cosy burnt. She said there was nothing like wool for carrying infection. I was surprised at this. According to my mother there was nothing like paper for carrying infection. If she got a letter from an infected area, however mild the infection and however distant the area, she would hold it gingerly between thumb and finger and put it in the oven to get a good baking. Often she would forget it was there and the correspondence was reduced to ash before she had become acquainted with its contents. If she heard there was scarlet fever about the newspapers were left to rot in the box down the lane where the paper-boy delivered them for us to collect. If the scarlet fever was rampant enough we could be without news for months.

When the measles were over I came out in a flourishing crop of carbuncles. They were extremely painful. They might not have been so painful if Mary hadn't been so angry with me for having them. Having measles in her nice clean sick bay was bad enough but the carbuncles added insult to injury. She had quite enough to do, she said, without having to rush around with hot fomentations for my carbuncles. She squeezed and fomented them with such ill-feeling that they grew and multiplied, instead of fading and dying in the shortest possible time.

On the day I took my first tottering steps back to the library Mr Chamberlain announced that a state of war existed between us and Germany, which, considering that it was slightly less than a year since he promised us it wouldn't, seemed a bit of a nerve on his part.

The news came as a shock to some and no surprise at all to others. For me it brought a kind of feverish excitement that I should be living in such stirring times. There was also a strong feeling of uncertainty about what tomorrow would bring forth. Until then, the next day, the next week, the next month had followed each other in a fairly predictable pattern. The biggest turmoil there had been in our lives was when we sat for our exams. Now all that was changed. Whatever lay before us had to be different from anything that was past.

Baker and Weldon heard the noise in stricken silence. There was no excitement in it for them, nor any pleasurable anticipation for what tomorrow might bring. There was only dread. Having new young husbands to worry about robbed war of all its cinematic glamour.

Davies was as stricken as they were. Though she had no husband, she had an Archibald. She saw nothing in the war that could bring him or her anything but unhappiness. I spent most of that first Sunday telling the others and myself that there was nothing to get either excited or depressed about. It would all be over by Christmas, I said.

The women heard the news and at first wouldn't believe it. Then they were angry, then they were sad. Then they started to look into the future, not liking what they saw. Some of them said it wouldn't last. Others knew it would and buried their heads in the pillows and wept.

The men were angry all the time. They'd seen it coming, they said. It should have come before, they said. It shouldn't have come at all, they said. But whatever they said, and however wise they chose to be after the event, it was upon us. But nothing went the way we expected it to go.

Part Two

Chapter Six

AFTER ALL THE fears and forebodings of an immediate holocaust the war got off to a slow start. Except for an early false alarm that had us scurrying to the trenches or rushing to assure the nervous that it was only a false alarm, nothing went as we had expected it to. This affected some in a curious way. Where were the air raids? the questioners asked, the poison gas, and the enemy invasion we'd been preparing for? And if there were to be none of these then why all the trench digging, the gas masks, and the children still being sent to safe areas with labels tied round their necks – and the elderly with their parrots and precious bits of porcelain, not to mention the expectant ladies with discreetly disguised bumps under their smocks who had been bundled into trains and hustled off to safety? 'Typical example of mismanagement by the high-ups,' said the typically uninformed vociferous know-alls. A.R.P. wardens and Civil Defence personnel grew tired of putting on their tin hats every night to go and sit in their posts playing brag, instead of rushing in bravely and heroically dragging out casualties from burning buildings as they had been training to do for a long time. They could have done with an air raid or two, they said, to liven things up a bit and give them a chance to get some practice in before they'd forgotten everything they'd ever learnt. The biggest thrill they got was when someone carelessly let a light shine under a door, or a beam escape from an ill-fitting black-out curtain. The local papers had long lists of these sinners with full reports of the remarks the magistrates had made when they sat on the Bench imposing the fines. The patients told us that the list caused a lot of suspicion among the neighbours. Allowing a light to flash brightly enough for a warden to notice was enough to lay the flasher open to a charge of indecently exposing the area to enemy attack. It could even have been deliberate – a flashed message to attract the attention of a secret agent. Nobody trusted anybody any more. There were spies everywhere, or so the rumour-spreaders would have had us believe.

But even we were astonished at the way things were going. Those of us who had dreamed of being heroines from the start found ourselves doing the daily round in exactly the same way as we had done it before the war broke out. The common task of giving out a bedpan was made no less common by the state of emergency that existed. The most important difference as far as we could see was that some of the chronics were being sent out.

This was so that their beds would be empty when patients more needful of them started pouring in. Getting them out had not always been easy. The tramps, hypochondriacs, and many others who had enjoyed ill health for a long time, often without the least trace of illness, were very upset when the doctors told them that the time had at last come for them to go back to the roads, to next-of-kin who didn't want them, or to the workhouse from which they had been admitted too long ago for any of us to remember the day. The man who had occupied a bed on one of the verandahs for years, suffering agonies from a complaint that only came on when someone suggested he should go home, was so taken aback by the doctors' firmness that he forgot to have an attack and went home almost without demur. His wife did all the demurring, but we wasted none of our sympathy on her. She'd had a long enough rest from his moaning while he was on the verandah doing his moaning at us.

There were some we didn't send home. One of these was Dummy, the deaf and dumb man on Male Two. He was far too valuable to us to be sent out even if there had been anywhere for us to send him to. Since the day he was admitted with a large hole in his throat he had become almost an integral part of the hospital. While he was around to grunt his advice to the nurses, and his censure of unruly patients it was reasonably certain that Male Two would survive whatever pressures endangered its survival.

But despite the anticlimax of a war that wasn't coming up to expectations there was still a strange feeling of excitement running through the hospital. It was strangely reminiscent of Christmas. At Christmas time the male nurses ran in and out of the female wards holding step-ladders for us to climb while we put up the decorations and balanced the fairy on top of the tree. But now they were in and out all the time, holding the steps and looking up our skirts while we fixed the blackout curtains, replaced light bulbs with ones that gave less light, and pasted strips of brown paper on the windows to ensure that they wouldn't get broken if a few tons of high explosive fell anywhere near them. The male nurses went away happy with the glimpses they'd been given of an inch of bare leg above stocking tops. It seemed that there might be some small compensation for being at war.

But we stopped feeling that there might be compensations when Baker's brother went down with his ship little more than a month after it all started. Instead we got a sudden premonition that this was just the beginning. Baker's brother had been a sailor long before the rumours of war had sent adventurous boys volunteering for the Navy rather than wait to be conscripted to the Army. He and I had walked through the snow one afternoon singing at the tops of our voices, and had walked back through it again quarrelling at the tops of our voices. We'd had some magnificent quarrels. We had hurled abuse, shouted insults, made it up then gone through it all again. When his leave was over and he went back to sea I missed his quarrels as much as I missed him. And now he was dead, and I couldn't believe it. But Baker believed it. She went home to comfort her parents and when she came back she told us that they also had believed it. From the things she said and the way she said them we gathered that the brief holiday had been no holiday at all.

For a while she was different. But not too different for very long. One day, after she had been looking through the library window, she turned to us and sighed. 'I suppose he's all right wherever he is,' she said. 'I just wish he wasn't at the bottom of the sea.' And so did I.

After that, except for giggling less and not wearing her pink hat with the daisies on it any more, she went back to being the Baker we knew. Though it was often remarked that she was kinder to the patients than she had been before; and she had always been kind to the patients. Thinking about it, we realized that it was her special way of coming to grips with things. A typical Baker way.

When Dr Collins went into the Air Force and Harry got his call-up papers for the Army we all went out for a fish and chip supper in the dirty little café we had been having fish and chip suppers in for years. It was not a jolly evening. Baker and Weldon were very quiet and Dr Collins and Harry had other things to think about than making bright chat over the cod. (Though Baker and Weldon were now married it would be a long time before their married names were bestowed upon them. Habit died hard and nobody was used to switching names while they were still working where they had been known by the old one.)

After Davies and I had said goodnight to the others outside the lodge gates we went to her room for a cigarette and talked about the evening. She suddenly became very thoughtful. 'They're different,' she said at last. I knew what she was talking about. I had realized that Baker and Weldon were different. It had shown in lots of little ways. I dwelt on it for a moment then came up with a brilliant explanation. 'It's because they're married, I expect,' I said. 'It's bound to show even though they are still only nurses.' I went blundering on. 'Why don't you and Archibald get married?' I asked, as if getting married was as simple as lighting our Woodbines. Davies sat and gazed down at the honey-combed counterpane on her bed. 'I would,' she said, 'but it's Archibald. He doesn't think it right for us to get married in wartime. He says supposing we had a baby and he wasn't there to see it.' I saw from her face that she knew exactly what he meant. Since Baker's brother had died we were only too aware of the dreadful things that could happen to people.

'But surely there doesn't have to be a baby,' I said

doubtfully. 'There must be ways. Think of Marie Stopes.' We thought of Marie Stopes. I also thought of all the women I had seen dying on Gynae because there didn't have to be a baby. When we had finished thinking we were still not much further forward. However good Marie Stopes may have been in her special field we had learned nothing about her field in the lecture room and had gleaned only the basics from other sources. Archibald didn't seem to know too much about it either.

We smoked one cigarette and were halfway through a second when Davies stubbed out hers and lit a third. I stared at her in horror. 'Waste not want not' was one of her favourite mottoes and neither of us was so well off that we could afford to stub out a cigarette when we were only halfway through it.

'Let's leave,' she said. 'We've passed our Finals and the others won't miss us now they've got husbands, so let's leave and go somewhere else.' I stubbed out my stub and searched frantically for the one she'd wasted. I took a long time relighting it before I said anything.

'Where would we go?' I asked at last. It was clear from the speed that she answered the question that she had been thinking about it for a long time.

'We'll go somewhere and get our T.B. Certificate,' she said, contemplating the counterpane again. If she hadn't looked so serious about it I would have laughed. Never once had Davies been sent on to the Sanatorium wards without looking into her handkerchief every time she coughed in search of blood. She was as certain of catching T.B. on the San. as the Irish girl had been of catching V.D. whenever she worked on the special clinic. She waited until I had finished telling her what I thought of the crazy idea then she went on as if I hadn't spoken.

'We could go to the sanatorium near London that Pickford went to when she left here.'

Pickford had left in a cloud of glorious disgrace while she was still doing her training. An ageing and jealous surgeon who had lusted after her for a long time saw her out one night with a more youthful doctor and waited for her on the drive, scalpel poised. Luckily nobody got hurt but Pickford had to go. We all knew it was the way she would have wanted to go. The only thing that would have improved the going for her would have been for the Sunday papers to feature it under banner headlines: '*Crime Passionnel.*' Pickford had made our dull days bright with her grossly exaggerated accounts of all the *crimes passionnels* she had provoked among her many boyfriends. When she last wrote to us from the Sanatorium where she had gone she was once more packing her bags. From her letter we could only assume that the Matron had inconsiderately appeared at the door while Pickford was giving some highly unorthodox treatment to a male patient in a bathroom. Since the hospital was strictly orthodox all other forms of treatment were frowned upon by the Matron. Pickford didn't seem too downhearted about it; she never did, she was a very resilient girl. We thought about her for a while then I asked Davies what had made her think of leaving. 'It's because of Archibald,' she said quietly. 'If I'm nearer London at least I'll be able to see more of him than I do now.' She didn't add that the time might come when she wouldn't be seeing him at all, but I knew that was what she meant.

We had never known what Archibald did in London. If Davies knew she never told us, and we never saw him in any sort of uniform at all. We puzzled over it and came to the conclusion that he was assigned to bigger things. We were right, but we didn't know for a long time how right we were.

The idea of going anywhere near London terrified me. The nearest I had ever been was when my school-teacher took me to the Wembley Exhibition, hoping that I might derive some cultural benefit from it. She hoped in vain. I cried all the way there and all the way back with plenty of hysterical shrieks in between. The thought of my mother back there in the depths of Lincolnshire and me in some foreign land thousands of miles away from her caused me unutterable grief. I tried telling this to Davies but she only snorted. 'You're older now,' she said truthfully. 'And I'd be with you.' As she said this it occurred to me that it must have taken a great deal of courage for her to make up her mind to go near London. London was a word, a place to be visited only in dreams. Those who boasted they had been to London were looked at in awe by those who had got no nearer to it than Stratford-on-Avon for a day's outing. And here she was, boldly suggesting that we should pack our bags and go there. I tried other ways of getting out of it. 'But what would my mother say?' I said, as helplessly as if I had been twelve instead of twenty-one. Davies snorted again.

'You're twenty-one and you can do as you like,' she said. 'And besides, you never go home now except on your holiday and you could still do that wherever we were. Your mother would hardly notice that you weren't still here.' I knew better. The fact that I was twenty-one wouldn't count at all with my mother. She didn't recognize such trifling landmarks. She made her own rules and just because somebody decreed that at twenty-one a girl could do as she liked didn't automatically mean that she had to agree with it. I anticipated a lot of difficulties arising when I told her I was leaving. I also anticipated difficulties when I mentioned London. My mother was an avid reader of the Sunday papers and kept herself informed about the things that went on in London, and though most of the things she read were totally outside her experience she would, I knew, put up a lot of resistance to my getting myself mixed up in them. I told Davies that I would think over all that she had said and let her know my decision in the morning.

By the time I had had a wash and got to bed I was too tired to think about anything, but in the morning I told Davies that I would leave and go with her to the sanatorium near London.

Chapter Seven

THE STORY OF our leaving had to be told to the others in two parts. From start to finish, with long intervals between the telling, it took a day. Davies began the first chapter while we were queuing for cocoa at first lunch. Since we had become staff-nurses we were granted the privilege of going to first mid-morning lunch, first dinner, tea and supper. The only advantage we got from the privilege was that there was marginally more food available. But if the amount was more generous the quality wasn't improved. By the time the end of the queue had reached the cocoa jug the drop that was left in it was thick with sediment.

'We're both leaving soon,' sang out Davies to Baker and Weldon who had pushed their way to the front of the queue. Being married had given them the confidence to do that kind of thing. Every nurse except them turned and stared at Davies. 'Leaving' was a drama that didn't happen often. Probationers became staff-nurses, staff-nurses became young sisters, and young sisters became old sisters; often cantankerous old sisters, far removed from the eager rosy-cheeked girls who had long ago aspired to become tender ministering angels.

Davies broadcast her news again and this time Baker and Weldon heard. They grabbed their cups and came back to us. 'What do you mean you're both leaving?' asked Weldon, staring at us as if we were mad.

'I mean we're both leaving,' said Davies, making the statement no more explicit than it was before.

'Where are you going?' asked Baker, wiping smears of undissolved cocoa from her mouth.

'We're going to the sanatorium Pickford went to after she left here,' answered Davies. Baker looked at her in horror.

'But that's not far away from London,' she said. 'You can't possibly go near London while there's a war on, you must both be out of your minds.' 'Stark raving mad,' chimed in Weldon.

Not having the courage or determination that Davies had I was inclined to agree with them; but I would have died rather than let them know I agreed with them. I was as vehement in the defence of our sanity as Davies was. United we might totter a little, but divided they would have made mincemeat of us.

That evening, instead of going straight home as they always did, Weldon and Baker skirted Mary who disapproved of non-residents paying calls on residents, and came across to my room. They sat on my bed while Davies and I gave them an outline of our plans for leaving. Because the plans we had made were still far from cut-and-dried we improvised on them as we went along, adding much that we hadn't thought of before and omitting much that we had. The omissions were mainly the snags. Baker was quick to see these for herself and lost no time in pointing them out to us.

'But why must you go to London?' she asked, when it had finally sunk in that we were going and no power on earth would stop us. No power on earth would have stopped Davies but I might have been stopped quite easily had I not committed myself so deeply that morning. Baker went on: 'Supposing they start bombing London as Granddad said they would, you could both be killed the moment you got there.' Davies was not to be swayed by such trifling considerations. Having made her bed and put her hand to the plough she was perfectly willing to lie down in the furrow, however high the risks. It wasn't in her nature to chop and change once she'd made up her mind about something. She explained about Archibald, and how she wanted to be near him until the time came when he might be far beyond her reach. When she had finished explaining they knew exactly what she meant. Baker would have done the same if it had brought her closer to Dr Collins and Weldon was only able to endure separation from Harry by the thought that he was stationed near enough to get home almost every weekend. They wasted no more time telling us we were mad. Instead, we sat and smoked and talked, until Baker thought of another small difficulty we might be up against when we got to London.

'How will you know what they're talking about?' she asked in her broad West Midland accent. 'They're all Cockneys down there, it'll be ages before you understand a word they're saying.' I remembered as she spoke that, according to the birth certificate my mother had produced the day before I went to be a nurse, I was born in London, and might even be a Cockney. I sprang loyally to the defence of Cockneys.

'They still speak English, even if they are Cockneys,' I said, a little huffily. 'And anyway, we're not going right into London, we shall only be on the outskirts. They perhaps aren't Cockneys as far out as that.' Baker said something about them all being Cockneys once you got past Coventry then she and Weldon said goodnight and went, tiptoeing with their shoes in their hands lest Mary had smelt a rat and was hovering somewhere – the 'rat' in this case being the cigarette smoke.

At ten o'clock the next morning Davies and I trembled together to the Matron's office. The thought of asking for permission to leave filled us with such terror that we stood for a long time on the corridor bracing ourselves for the ordeal, and allowing others behind us in the queue to precede us into the office. This they regarded as a doubtful privilege: they also needed time for bracing.

When we could no longer put off the evil moment we gave ourselves a final brace, took a deep breath and plunged through the door. The Matron looked up sharply. Seeing nurses in twos wasn't the accepted custom. She sensed from our united front that the visit portended more than a simple request for a sleeping-out pass. She offered no help with the preambles and even the dog looked startled and forgot to snarl. I stepped back a few inches in order to establish that it was Davies who had the lead part and I was only there as her understudy.

When Davies had finished saying what had to be said she died down and the Matron spent a little time examining the surface of her desk. After she had satisfied herself that the veneer was up to specified standard she began to speak. What she said surprised me. I had expected thunderbolts. There were none.

'But why a sanatorium, Nurse?' she asked. She had obviously heard through the grapevine about Davies's anxiety neurosis whenever she was put on a San. ward and was as puzzled about it as I was.

'Please, Matron,' said Davies, stammering slightly for the first time. 'I – we – she, well, we thought it might be a good idea if we went somewhere and got our T.B. Certificates. We – she – I thought it would come in useful sometime.' Though Davies wasn't to know it then, they never did come in useful for we never got them. The war had other plans for us. The Matron gave her desk a further inspection then she looked up and inspected me.

'And what about you, Nurse?' she said. 'Are you in favour of this idea?'

'Yes, Matron,' I said bravely, goaded to bravery by the threatening look Davies gave me. The Matron turned back to the chief spokeswoman.

'Very well, Nurse,' she said, doing some furious scribbling on a desk jotter. 'Since it seems reasonably certain that hostilities will cease within the next few months I see no good reason why you should not both be allowed to leave. You may proceed with your arrangements.' As hostilities had still not properly begun we got the permission we sought under an entirely false premise, but at least we got it. The dog waddled across to us, sniffed up Davies's skirt and round my ankles and we left the office. We were drained of energy. Despite the number of visits we had paid her over the years, a visit to the Matron had lost none of its terrors.

When all the usual letter writing had been done and the Matron of the sanatorium had finally agreed to accept us we went back to the office and cravenly begged for the annual leave we were entitled to and which was overdue. We used it to go home and break the news to our mothers that we were leaving our training school and going to a sanatorium near London.

The journey home took a long time for me: almost twice as long as it had taken when there were no troop trains rattling past to shunt us into sidings, and no ammunition trucks to channel us into cuttings. At each delay windows were lowered and heads stuck out while passengers complained furiously at the delay. The nervous types jumped to nervous conclusions about bombs on the line and invaders in the bushes. After they were assured by the less nervous that none of these things were happening their nervousness turned to anger and they joined in the general complaining. They were happy at having something to complain about to take their mind off their fears.

I had nothing to complain about. I had never enjoyed a journey home so much in my life. Before, whenever I had gone home, the train had been full of farmers' wives taking their eggs and butter to sell in the busy little market town, and their bucolic husbands haggling over fat stock prices. Now all that was changed. The carriage I was in still had its sprinkling of locals, but there was a much heavier sprinkling – amounting almost to a shower – of servicemen and their kitbags. The kitbags took up so much room that we were having to put our feet up on them to make room for more passengers to get in and squeeze us to death. I found myself wedged between a soldier and an airman which was far more interesting than sharing a seat with a crate of day-old chicks. The pressures caused by the wedging became extremely pleasurable sometimes, especially when we swayed dangerously round bends or groped our way through dark tunnels. The delights of the groping and swaying were shared equally between the airman, the soldier and me.

On several platforms on the route we saw the evacuees that Baker had told us about. They looked just as sad as she said they did. They stood in forlorn little groups clutching gas masks and teddy bears while teachers and wardens and women in drab green uniforms bustled about organizing them. There were a few mothers crying, and some fathers trying not to cry. I was glad when the train rumbled past the smallholding where my parents lived, and came to a halt at the little station down the long lane. I foolishly thought that here was one place that war couldn't possibly have touched.

My mother's letters had always been brief. They said only the things that were uppermost in her mind while she was writing them. One of her most recent had brought me bad news. 'Hope this finds you well as it leaves us at present,' I read. 'Except for your father's lumbago and the old horse dying.' The old horse had been dying for a long time. It was kept out of charity in the paddock near the house. It ended its days in the gorse bushes beside the railway track. My mother went on to assure me that it had died peacefully and begged me not to fret. She told me to 'keep smilling', and enclosed a postal order for two and sixpence to enable me to keep smilling. My mother's spelling had never been perfect.

So, though I was prepared for there being no horse in the paddock, I was entirely unprepared for what there was. The field was alive with soldiers. Instead of the peace I expected there was war all around me. I stood looking at the gun emplacements and the searchlights, scarcely able to believe my eyes.

My mother had told the soldiers that I was on the way. The news of my arrival spread through the gorse bushes like wildfire and within seconds I had a whole battery of men rushing to take my suitcase off me and relieve me of my umbrella. From the eager way they volunteered for the duties I could only assume they had been without home leave for a long time. I should have felt flattered but I didn't. All I felt was the deepest sympathy for them. I knew only too well that the place where I lived, and where they had the misfortune to be stationed, was so lacking in females below the age of middle that I must have dropped as manna from heaven. Alas, they didn't know my mother as well as I did. I knew there wasn't the slightest chance of her allowing me free range among the gorse bushes. She was already standing at the kitchen door, waiting to grab me from the hands of love-starved soldiers. Any hopes they may have nurtured of sating their hunger on me were quickly dashed. I could only hope they knew that it was my mother who was doing the dashing and not me. Given the chance I would gladly have taken at least the edge off their appetites.

When I was safely in the kitchen and the preliminary greetings were over I looked around in amazement.

'Whatever's that?' I asked, pointing to the monstrosity that had taken root under the window. My mother followed my eyes.

'It's a sink,' she said.

I went across to it. 'But it looks like a horse trough,' I said, examining it.

'It is a horse trough,' she said. 'That's why it looks like one.'

'Then what's it doing in here?' I asked.

'It's our new sink,' she said, gazing at it with fondness in her eyes.

'I thought you said it was a horse trough,' I reminded her.

'Well, it is a horse trough,' she replied. 'But after the old horse died the soldiers brought it in and turned it into a sink. I forgot to mention it in my letter.' I looked closely at the newly installed piece of equipment, taking in its finer points, or lack of them.

'But there's no outlet for the dirty water,' I said at last. For as long as I could remember we had washed ourselves and the dirty dishes in a bowl on the kitchen table and thrown the dirty water into a brook that ran beside the house. The method was simple and foolproof, except when it was raining, then we allowed the dirty water to accumulate in a bucket under the table and emptied it when the weather improved. It would have been a waste of time and energy to put on a pair of wellington boots and a raincoat just to empty a bowl of water. My mother started to go a faint puce colour.

'If all you've come home for is to pick holes in things the sooner you go back the better,' she retorted angrily. I apologized to her for picking holes in things and went back to scrutinizing the horse trough. It was perched on top of a badly built brick plinth. The hole that had originally drained it off was now blocked up with a large quantity of the cement that had been used to adhere the bricks together. I noticed suddenly that there were no taps.

'But there are no taps,' I said to my mother.

'There never were,' she answered, with truth.

'But we didn't need them while we were using the bucket and bowl,' I said. 'What good is a sink without taps?' My mother began to swell with anger again. Again I apologized.

'All right then,' I said, abandoning the taps, 'but how do you get the water in and out of it?' My mother looked at me in despair. I had obviously learnt nothing since I left home. Certainly nothing in the way of commonsense.

'We fetch the hot water in a ladle out of the boiler next to the fire, then we pour it into the sink. When the water's dirty we scoop it out with the ladle and throw it in the brook the same as we always did.' She gave the horse trough a friendly pat.

'But surely you're no better off than you were before?' I said, risking her anger again.

'Of course we are,' she said, the puce showing again. 'We've got a sink now what we never had before.' I could see that the soldiers had opened up new horizons for my parents and given them a taste of modern living. My mother led me into the living-room.

'They give us stuff as well,' she said, modestly lowering her eyes.

'What sort of stuff?' I asked.

'All sorts of stuff,' she said. 'Things like sugar and tea, and tinned salmon and fruit.' She threw open the bookcase door and revealed a store of sugar and tea, tinned salmon and a variety of tinned fruit. The set of *Children's Encyclopaedia* that Santa Claus had brought me when I was eight had been removed to make way for the groceries, as had *Pilgrim's Progress*, *Gulliver's Travels* and all the other literary gems that had stayed in the bookcase unread for years. I could see that if the time ever came for official rationing to start it would cause less hardship to my mother while the soldiers were stocking the bookcase. Much later, when spivs and black marketeers were being reviled by the righteous I kept quiet. Having parents living on tinned salmon, with mixed fruit salad to follow, the whole washed down with endless cups of well-sweetened tea put me in no position to join in the reviling.

The excitement of finding the soldiers in the paddock and the horse trough in the kitchen had temporarily taken my mind off the tidings I had come to bring. I had still said nothing about the move to the sanatorium when my father got in from work. He looked pleased to see me, though he didn't say much. He was a quiet man, never saying two words if he thought one would suffice. I waited until he was settled in his wooden armchair and had lit his pipe before I opened my mouth to speak – but it was my mother who spoke.

'We're getting some evacuees next week,' she said, laying a clean cloth on the table. My father took the pipe out of his mouth, gazed at its dying embers and applied another dozen matches to it. When the sitting-room was aswirl with smoke he looked through it at my mother. 'How many?' he asked, as calmly as if getting some evacuees was a thing that was happening to them all the time.

'I said two,' my mother told him. 'But I promised that if things started getting bad we'd have another couple.' My father nodded approvingly and puffed contentedly for a moment or two. Then he looked at me.

'It'll get worse, Birdie,' he said. 'It'll get a lot worse yet.' Birdie was the name he used whenever he needed a name for me. 'And when it does,' he went on, 'them bairns in the towns will need somewhere safe to go.' I looked from him to my mother and marvelled. Years ago, when we lived on a farm, we had taken two children throughout the summer as part of a Country Holiday scheme. I remembered them well. They had so thoroughly disorganized everything that when the holiday was ended it took my mother weeks to get things back the way she liked them to be. And here she was, no longer young, offering her home to children who would no doubt climb into the pigsty, fall off the haystack, and smear her shining brass and gleaming steel with their sticky fingers – all things that I was never allowed to do when I was a child. I gave her a warm look.

The look embarrassed her so much that she jumped to defend herself against a charge of softness.

'When them Nazis start dropping their bombs on places it'll be London and the big towns they'll go for first,' she said slamming a teapot on the table. I seized the opening.

'I'm leaving the hospital and going to a sanatorium near London to get my T.B. Certificate,' I burst out. There was a sudden stillness. My father took his pipe out of his mouth and did things with tobacco and my mother stood for a moment with a bundle of knives and forks in her hand. Then she laid them on the table and turned to get the cups and saucers off the dresser. I noticed she got the best ones that were only usually used when we had visitors, or at Christmas. It was a long time before she stopped rattling the crockery. When she did she stood with both hands on my father's chair.

'She'd better look after herself when she gets to London,' she said, brushing a strand of hot tobacco off the front of my father's shirt. 'There's a lot of funny folk down there.' My father nodded. 'And mind you keep your chest wrapped up,' she said to me. 'You don't want to go catching consumption. You was always a bit bronichal when you was a baby.' And that was all that was said about my going to London. War was already making distance nearer and sin less important. My mother had been as much concerned with me catching consumption as she was about me catching the more deadly ills that were hinted at in the Sunday papers. I spent a short while assuring her that nurses didn't catch things, trying, as I assured her, not to think of all nurses who had caught things since nursing first began. Though we were taught by our sister-tutor to believe that catching things was the result of carelessness and seldom an accident things were still caught, and often the worst sort of things, like tuberculosis for example.

My mother seemed reassured by my reassurance. Any fears she may have had of my expiring at an early age with galloping consumption were apparently allayed. She relayed the assurance to my father and he smoked his pipe contentedly until tea was ready.

Most of my week's holiday was spent getting ready for the evacuees. I helped my mother boil the bedspreads, beat the carpets, take mothballs out of blankets and whitewash the back bedroom ceiling. And all the time we worked I listened longingly to the comings and goings which were an indication that the soldiers had been forewarned of the arrival of the evacuees and were making provision for feeding the extra mouths. They may also have been an indication that the soldiers were trying to force me out of the glasshouse my mother was keeping me in. If so their efforts met with no success.

The evacuees arrived on the last day of my holiday. They were two unhappy, travel-stained little girls, clinging to each other for comfort. They also clung to their gas masks, the labels round their necks and a lot of small toys in a carrier bag. These were the things their mother had sent them off with and they had no intention of letting two strange women take them from them. My mother tried coaxing and I tried comforting. It was all to no avail. Their tears still fell.

I took them out to see the pigs but they didn't like pigs. I showed them the fowls but they were terrified of fowls. I allowed them to peer down the well but that sent them off into hysterical shrieks. Nothing made up for not having their mother with them.

When my father came home he solved the problem at once. He blew their noses on his red and white spotted handkerchief, spruced up their labels and led them out of the house, each holding tightly to a work-gnarled hand. As they went I heard him talking to them. 'Come along, my Birdies,' I heard him say. 'Come with me to look at the guns and talk to the soldiers in the field.' They went happily. They knew about guns, they were springing up like mushrooms in the place they had come from. They knew about soldiers, their father was one. Pigs and fowls and deep dark wells were part of the strange land they had so cruelly been banished to.

When it was time for me to go I went a little sadly. Hearing my father bestow his pet name for me on the evacuees had sparked off a small flame of jealousy and I would have liked more interest shown in my amazing courage at going near to London in wartime. Neither of my parents waved to me as I walked down the cart-track; they were taken up at the time with something the evacuees were doing. But the soldiers waved, and I thought there was a slight wistfulness about their waving. They had pinned a lot of hopes on me and they were no better off when I went than they were when I arrived. I waved back to them and went on down the lane.

Davies told me that her mother had been terribly impressed about us going to London. She had warned Davies to make sure she wasn't taken advantage of, saying that it was the easiest thing in the world for a girl to be taken advantage of in London. As far as I know Davies was never taken advantage of, and neither was I. Though the prospect didn't daunt me as much as it did her.

The preparations for leaving our training school were less worrying than the preparations for going there had been. Without my mother to guide me I bought things I desired rather than things I required. Davies and I both treated ourselves to a pair of French knickers, wide-legged and immoral. We squandered money on art silk stockings, and frittered more away on slinky nightdresses to replace the winceyette tents our mothers had forced us into. With the coppers that were left after the indulgences were paid for and our tickets bought in advance we got a few cigarettes to repay those we owed, and then faced weeks of poverty until payday came round again.

On the day we went Baker and Weldon came to the station to see us off. They were gratifyingly tearful at the thought of our going and waved to us until the train turned a bend and we could no longer see them waving.

If they had waited there another hour they could have done the farewell scene all over again.

Chapter Eight

THE TRAIN THAT took us to London, from where we were to get another to the sanatorium, was packed even tighter than the one I had travelled home in. Kitbags were piled high and precariously, threatening all the time to descend from overhead racks and crash down on somebody's skull. Passengers who had been crafty enough, tough enough or frail enough to get themselves a seat were glared at angrily, deliberately tripped over or spitefully kicked in the shins by passengers who were having to stand. There were no corridors and consequently no lavatories or anything as luxurious as a restaurant, or even a dirty buffet car. There was a complete lack of anything that could be called comfort. The only comfort we had was the comfort of knowing that we were at last on our way to London. Even this comfort was soon to be denied us.

We had been jolting along at a steady pace for what seemed like a long time when the landscape started taking on a familiar look. Sights that had been pointed out and silently said goodbye to suddenly began to loom up again. Slowly we steamed back into the station we had so recently steamed out of.

As we clanked to a halt on the platform civil war broke out. Furious soldiers, fuming airmen, seething sailors and extremely irate civilians waved their fists in the air and asked each other and the harassed porters what was going on. None of the passengers had any inside information and if the porters knew anything they were keeping it to themselves. The train now standing on platform five remained there for a long time. It occasionally gave a lurch as if making up its mind to move, then thought better of it, pulled up sharply and stayed where it was. None of us dared to get out and stretch our legs or do things like washing our hands in case somebody annexed the sitting or standing room we had managed to acquire.

After a long time and another hundred or two passengers we started getting up steam again, but not before the porters had reminded us rudely and often that we could expect inconveniences like no conveniences, and circular tours that took an hour to circle. There was a war on, they said, in case any of us had forgotten. None of us had.

When at last the train whistled and belched its way out of the station there were no Baker and Weldon to wave to us and wish us a pleasant journey.

The journey was a great deal more pleasant than we had expected it to be. It took a few miles to break down our inborn British reticence but once it was broken down everybody started to behave in a most unBritish way. The soldiers talked to us, we talked to the airmen, and the sailors talked to the civilians in almost endless permutation. The people who were sitting offered their knees to those who were standing, and the girls who were standing at first blushed and refused the knees, then they decided that anything might be better than having to stand all the way to London. Soon there were far fewer standing.

When somebody complained of feeling hungry sandwiches were brought out and exchanged for bars of chocolate, apples were halved and oranges quartered. Flasks were drained to the last drop to let everybody in the carriage enjoy a mouthful. The delays on the way were taken in good part and when it began to get dark the blinds were pulled down and a small blue light that gave hardly any light at all came on, throwing eerie shadows over everything and turning healthy faces into ghastly masks. The shadows became a screen for one or two attempted passes that hadn't been mentioned in the servicemen's travel warrants but anything that looked like getting out of control was quickly contained by a warning cough from one of the more senior travellers. We were glad when we finally reached London but ready to admit that the journey could have been a lot worse than it had been.

The dingy, dimly lit terminus we steamed into was as

packed with people as the train had been. There were masses of servicemen and mounds of kitbags everywhere. Yet, in spite of the milling throng, a curious silence hung over the station, reminding us of church. Nobody seemed to be talking in a normal voice. Except for the noise of trains gathering strength to move out and others dissipating their energies moving in, all noise was muted. Couples saying goodbye said it hardly above a whisper, and couples saying hello said it almost as softly. The station was the most depressing place I had ever been in.

Davies and I stood about for a while hoping that somebody would notice us and ask if we needed any help, but nobody did. Everybody was too busy arranging their own lives to be able to spare time for arranging ours. At last Davies spoke, but only in a whisper.

'We were told to look for an underground train or something,' she said, looking vaguely round in search of one. There was nothing in sight that remotely resembled an underground train. Neither of us had ever seen one but we were sure it would have differences that marked it out from the ordinary sort. Then Davies darted into the shadows and I heard her talking to somebody. I shrank back, remembering the warnings her mother had given her about being taken advantage of. Suddenly the prospect lacked any allurement. When she returned she had a man with her.

'You shouldn't have spoken to him,' I hissed. 'He's a strange man and he could be anybody for all we know.'

'He's a porter,' she hissed back at me. 'And if we don't ask somebody we'll be here all night.' The porter waited patiently while we discussed the possibility of him being a white slave trafficker. He was a fatherly sort of man and realized the dilemma we were in. He perhaps had daughters of his own at home. When we finally decided to trust him he led us down some stairs and showed us where the underground trains were. Then he left us.

It was after we had bought our tickets and got through the turnstiles that we came up against the next obstacle. It was an obstacle that even Baker hadn't warned us about. Probably it was one she didn't know about. Immediately in front of us there was a staircase that caterpillared its way to the bowels of the earth. Davies and I put our cases down and stared at it. Neither of us had seen one before. I turned to her.

'You're not getting me on that thing,' I said. 'Wild horses wouldn't drag me on it. There must surely be some proper stairs for us to walk down.' I was prepared to walk for ever rather than be conveyed by such a terrible conveyor belt.

'No, there aren't,' said Davies. 'The underground trains are halfway down to Australia and it would take hours to get there on ordinary stairs.' I wasn't to be moved.

I was still standing there arguing with her when two airmen drew up alongside and dumped their kitbags next to our luggage.

'Go on,' said one of them, giving me a push in the back. 'It's all right once you get started. All you have to do is put one foot on, then the other and you're off.' He swung his kitbag over his shoulder and was away.

'Try it,' said the other airman. I did, and before I knew where I was I had been carried away by the staircase.

Getting off required as much courage as getting on, but with the help of the airman who had got there before me I staggered off the bottom step and fell into his arms. I remained there until Davies arrived. She got off without any help at all, which was only to be expected. She was an extremely well-balanced girl.

When we told the airmen where we were going they told us that the R.A.F. camp they were stationed at was in the same town as the Sanatorium. This sounded very promising to me. A town with an R.A.F. camp in it was exactly what I needed. I was twenty-one and past my first youth, and with no ring on my finger and no bottom drawer I was looking for something to get me out of a rut. There had been a long period of stagnation in my love life.

While we were waiting for the train to come in the airmen talked to us. The things they said threw new light on the war that was dragging its feet. They made the Matron's optimism about hostilities ceasing in the next few months seem suddenly ridiculous. Hitherto Davies and I had half believed those who said it would all be over almost before it started but listening to the things the airmen were saying made us have second thoughts.

One of them looked round the dreary cavern that was the underground station. 'It'll come in nice and handy for an air-raid shelter when they start bombing London,' he said cheerfully. We looked to see if he was joking and saw that he wasn't. But even he couldn't have known how short a time it would be before the cavern became a grim and fearful air-raid shelter.

When the train drew to a smooth standstill on the platform it had all its windows pasted over with anti-blast material, except for a spy-hole in the middle that was too small to see through. Because it was dark, and the stations were unlit and unnamed we had no idea where we where. The airmen told us that the secret was to count the stations as we stopped at them. They did the counting for us and soon we were again standing on a platform. This time above ground.

When we asked a porter where we could get a bus to the hospital he sounded very cross. And where, he asked, did we think we could get a bus at that time of night? Wasn't there enough trouble getting drivers already, without people like us wanting buses to run all night? It was still not quite nine o'clock. We apologized for asking and started trudging away with our baggage. The airmen said that if we didn't mind they were going the same way and would see us safely to the hospital. We didn't mind at all.

It had occurred to me while the porter was telling us off that in spite of what Baker had said about us not understanding a word once we got south of the Midlands I understood perfectly all that the porter had said. I also understood why he had said it. He was cold and tired, and fed up with the war and the inconveniences it was causing. He was even more fed up with people like us who demanded impossible things like buses that ran after nine o'clock at night. Though hostilities hadn't yet properly started, there was enough hostility about to set people's nerves on edge. It was only when hostilities began in earnest that everybody became comrades in adversity. Or almost everybody. There were always a few exceptions.

The road to the hospital was long and dark. We were very glad of the airmen's company. In the distance we could see searchlights criss-crossing the sky, and once we heard the sound of a plane approaching. A searchlight sprang to life quite near to us and picked out the silver streak of the plane. Then the sound died away and we were in the dark again.

At the hospital gates the airmen thankfully unloaded our luggage on to us. We thanked them very much; they said not at all, it had been a pleasure; they said they hoped they'd see us in the town sometime; we said we hoped so too; then we all stood in embarrassed silence until they walked away and left us to our fate.

Our immediate fate was a lodgeman. He peered suspiciously at us, in the time-honoured fashion of all lodgemen, then, not able to see all he wanted to see through the half-raised flap of his blackout curtain, he came out of the lodge and shone a small torch on our faces. When he had satisfied himself that if we were the enemy we were at least enemy women and not enemy men, he asked us who we were and why we were there. It took time and patience before we had completely established our identity. He was a man who, far from expecting hostilities to cease in the near future, clearly foresaw the day when the country would be overrun with enemy agents and he had no intention of allowing one to penetrate his defences. We respected him for his diligence. We knew it would be dictators like him who would save the country from foreign dictatorship. He gave us another quick interrogation then told us where we would find the night-sister. She took a lot of finding.

The hospital was small but extended over a wide area. We went over a lot of ground several times before we came upon the night-sister. When we did she was an entirely new experience. She was young and not at all frightening. She talked to us as if we were human beings and not nurses at all. This, coming on top of a tiring day, was almost too much for us to adjust to. We would have felt more at home with a bit of fuming and fury.

She took us across to a nurses' home that even in the dark looked very new, though the sandbags that were stacked up against the walls hid most of it. The room she led us to amazed us by its opulence. It was more of a hotel than a nurses' bedroom. Instead of iron bedsteads there were low wooden divans, instead of woodwormy wardrobes there were built-in cupboards, and in place of cold lino there was a carpet. It all looked very rich.

The sister apologized for the double room but explained that because of the war, Civil Nursing Reserves and Auxiliary nurses had started coming in. This put a strain on the accommodation. She told us that we would be asked to become non-resident as soon as possible to ease the problem of overcrowding in the home. After telling us more that we needed to know and asking if there was anything else we required she went. Neither of us had dared to tell her we were hungry. Within minutes she was back, apologizing for not asking if we were hungry. The apology almost ruined our appetites for the array of food she brought. We were entirely unused to sisters apologizing to nurses for anything, and certainly not for forgetting to feed them. We were just as unused to having food brought to us in bed by a sister.

While we ate she talked to us. She told us that many

of the sanatorium patients had been sent home, leaving only those who for various reasons weren't fit to be sent anywhere. She said the beds were being kept empty ready for when the bomb casualties and wounded servicemen started coming in. Just as the airmen had she made it sound as if war was waiting round the corner ready to spring.

Before she gathered up the tray and said goodnight she reminded us that we were to report to the Matron at nine-thirty in the morning. Because we had had such a tiring journey, she said, we didn't have to go on duty until after the Matron had seen us. It was all vastly different from the day I first started my training. That day nobody had even remembered to tell me where the lavatory was.

After the night-sister had gone Davies and I tried to stay awake long enough to talk but we were asleep before we had even got as far as Baker and Weldon waving us off at the station. It had indeed been a tiring journey.

Part Three

Chapter Nine

IF THE TREATMENT we got from the night-sister had shaken our confidence the cup of tea that was brought to us the next morning before we got up was enough to unnerve us completely. I had never drunk a cup of tea in bed in my life. My mother hadn't believed in such idle extravagances. The kitchen, she said, was the place for eating and drinking, or the living-room should there be visitors. The bedroom, she insisted, was a place for sleeping in and never meant to be used as a restaurant, nor would be in her house while folks had the strength to walk downstairs. The home-sister at our training school had echoed her sentiments. However sick we felt when we were in sick bay we were expected to heave ourselves out of bed at meal-times and sit respectably at a table. If we weren't well enough to get out of bed we weren't well enough to eat. Or so said Mary.

None but the most senior of ward sisters was allowed breakfast in bed, and then only once a month on their day off. On that auspicious occasion the most junior nurse on the ward was assigned to the task of 'doing the sister's breakfast'. It was a tremendous responsibility. She assembled an indifferently boiled egg, a slice of cold and rubbery toast, a dab of patients' marge and a cup of pallid tea, threw it all on to a cheap tin tray and bore it across to the honoured one. And here were we, still only staff nurses, getting a cup of tea brought to us in bed.

The girl who brought it was no longer a girl. She wore a white coat bedecked with blue epaulettes. The uniform was so far removed from anything we had ever seen a nurse wearing that at first we thought she must be the cook. When we asked her as tactfully as we could what exactly she was, she told us loftily that she was not the cook, she was a member of the Civil Nursing Reserve and was only working because there was a war on. Without the war she would be at home, putting her feet up in the afternoon, or writing long letters to her family scattered round the country. We begged her pardon for thinking she was the cook. She forgave us and told us where the dining-room was. Breakfast was at eight, she told us. More luxury. Breakfast had been at seven at our training school.

We drank the tea feeling very sinful. Almost from the cradle Davies and I had been taught to know our places and tea in bed was definitely above our station.

While we were drinking it Davies looked across at me from the mod. con. of her bed.

'What are we supposed to wear to go to breakfast and to see the Matron?' she asked. I had wondered the same myself. The first difference we noticed when we filled in the application papers for the new job was that there was no mention of uniform. We worried about it and wrote letters about it. Then we were told that we were not to worry, our uniform was an emolument like our food and washing, and would be provided free. When I thought of the sacrifices my mother had made to send me off to be a nurse with six of these and six of those and several pairs of the others, I realized that nursing was moving very slightly in a different direction. The movement was snail-like, and there would be a lot of hold-ups on the way, but at least there was movement.

I lay for a moment, baffled by the problem of what we should wear.

'Well,' I said at last. 'We haven't any uniform, we couldn't wear our nightdresses so it will have to be our best dresses.' We went down to breakfast feeling very conspicuous in our best dresses.

When we got back to the bedroom Davies started peeling off her stockings.

'I daren't go to the Matron in coloured stockings,' she said, rummaging in a drawer for a pair of black ones. I knew how she felt. I had not been seen by a Matron in anything but full uniform since the day I started my training. There seemed something quite wrong in appearing before her in a floral dress with cap sleeves. I also changed my stockings and put on a cardigan to cover my arms. The stockings and the cardigan lent a more official look to our best dresses – or so we hoped.

The Matron was another new experience. She was not at all like the Matron we had known and feared before. She was smaller and younger and had no snarling dog to sniff up our skirts. Her greeting threw me off balance as much as the moving staircase had. First she asked us if we had slept well and seemed genuinely interested in the answer. Then she apologized for there being no uniform waiting for us in our room. She explained that the war was disorganizing everything, even the sewing room. So many of the girls had left to join the Wrens, Waafs and A.T.S. that only skeleton staffs remained to shorten aprons and let out dresses. She told us the rules, making them sound less rule-like than the ones we'd obeyed – or not – over the years. This was an illusion. They needed just as much skill to circumvent as the others had. Then she brought the interview to an end by saying she hoped we'd be very happy working at the hospital. We left the office feeling as if we hadn't been to the Matron at all.

'She's funny, isn't she?' I said to Davies when we got out. I remembered my mother saying there were some funny folk in London, but I hadn't expected to come across one quite so soon, especially as we were not even in London but only on the outskirts.

'She's certainly different,' said Davies cautiously. She never made hasty judgements. She took time to form an opinion and once it was formed she stuck by it. Unlike me who loved or hated on sight then had an almost immediate change of heart, thus putting a severe strain on every new attachment I made.

'What do you think she meant when she said she hoped we'd be happy working at the hospital?' I asked, desperately seeking for a hidden meaning behind the simple courtesy. Davies thought about it for a moment.

'She probably meant she hopes we'll be happy working at the hospital,' she said, making it sound so simple. I wished I could be as trusting. For a Matron to hope such a thing and put the hope into words filled me with deep suspicion. There had to be a catch in it somewhere. Only after the final tuck had been taken out of my uniform dresses in the sewing room was I willing to admit that Davies might be right and the Matron really had hoped we'd be happy working at the hospital. It was very unsettling for me. I liked things the way they had always been. Any departure from the norm threw me into an agony of doubt, and still does.

Our new hospital stood on the brow of a hill with fields on one side, woods the other and a village little pub at the end of one of the fields. Like our paddock at home, the fields were strewn with soldiers, guns and searchlights. Above it all, billowing and buffeting in the wind, hung a silver barrage balloon. It was the first I had seen and its huge shape made me think again of what the airmen had said while we waited for the underground train. The prospect of an early peace took several steps back.

Anything even remotely vulnerable to attack was protected with layers of sandbags and wherever there had once been a grassy patch there was now a trench dug deep enough to give shelter in an emergency, until more permanent shelters were built. Though we were well away from the huddle of London it seemed that nobody was taking any chances.

From the top of the hill I caught a glimpse of the buildings that had housed the Wembley Exhibition and, remembering the anguish the visit there had caused me, I felt a little homesick just looking at it.

I was sent to Female Surgery and Davies to the Male side. The medical wards were almost empty. The patients who were fit enough had been sent home and told to go to their local T.B. clinics for regular check-ups and any minor treatment they might need. But there were enough patients left on the Surgical side to keep us busy. Since most of them were in spinal beds or making slow recovery from major chest surgery they needed long hospitalization. This meant that there was more for us to do than tend to their physical needs. Most of them were very unhappy as well as very ill.

The women resented their long stay in hospital while there was a war on. Most of them were Londoners and most of them came from parts of London that were over-populated and over-industrialized. They knew only too well from the preparations that were being made for aerial warfare that if it came it would be concentrated on the docks and factories that were the view they got from their windows at home. They disliked having only one lung instead of two, or less than their proper share of ribs since some had been removed. They longed to be with their families, sharing trouble and facing unknown peril. They grieved when their children were packed off to safety in the country when they were not there to do the packing. The doctors spent a lot of time giving them good reasons why they couldn't go home. There was at least one battle a day.

'No, you can't go home. You know you can't. You're not nearly well enough yet.'

'I never shall be well enough, lying here worrying me guts out about them at home.'

'You need at least another month.'

'Make it a week.'

'We'll see how you are in a fortnight.' But long before the fortnight was over the battle raged again. From the moment the women were allowed up to totter to the bathroom on our arm they were insisting they could just as easily be tottering to their own bathroom at home, if there was such a luxury as a bathroom at home. They were discharging themselves all the time against advice, willing to die with a collapsed lung rather than be in hospital when the buildings started to collapse around their families. The doctors were often powerless to stop them.

Davies said the men were just as difficult. They had more to worry about than the constant worry of wives and children. Being tubercular in peacetime was bad enough, with nothing but a bit of relief money coming in, plus a shilling or two the wife earned doing washing for the wealthy. But being tubercular in wartime had its own special problems. It was a blow to the pride as well as to the pocket. The men who could get out of bed sat beside those who couldn't. They played cards and talked. Most of the talk was lies.

'Bloody glad I'm in here and not out there,' one of them would say laying down his royal flush. 'Me brother volunteered last week. Catch me going before they sent for me.' And the others would look suspiciously at the royal flush and agree wholeheartedly that to volunteer rather than wait to be called up was the height of folly. There wasn't one of them who wouldn't rather have volunteered than be stuck in a sanatorium while there was a war on. But it didn't do to let everybody know how it felt to be a consumptive in wartime. The men played cards, embroidered tablecloths, and made wickerwork trays as if the occupational therapy was as beneficial to the war effort as it was supposed to be for them.

The village little pub on the corner was strictly out of bounds for the patients, which made it all the more enticing to go to. With plenty of friendly cooperation from those who weren't on graded walks those who were could often upgrade the walks before the doctor did, and make them stretch as far as the pub; or even dodge the sister or the chief male nurse in charge of Male San. and nip out across the field in the evening. The pub, the field and the surrounding woods offered more scope for romance than many of them would have got at home – especially the married ones. Dewy-eyed girls, and boys flushed with success, came in late for meals and late for bed, shielded by false evidence from their bed-bound friends. Suspicious nurses looked the other way unless there was enough reason to voice their suspicions.

When most of the ambulant patients had gone home there was less demand for the glasses and tankards that the landlord of the pub kept separately from the others as a precaution against his healthy customers catching more than a taste for beer from the less healthy ones. But if the special trade had fallen off the regular trade got a boost when the soldiers arrived and started making it their 'local'. It was then that the girls from the Female San. stopped pining for the boys who had vanished from the Male San. They found plenty of consolation in the woods and the fields.

The new romances caused more trouble than the old ones had. Most inter-sanatorium relationships owed their continued success to equally graded walks and a great many other things being equal. They could come to a sudden and unilateral end when one of the participants either got better and went home, or became worse and had to be confined to bed. This happened so often that it seldom caused inconsolable grief. It was a hazard that had to be faced if you were a T.B. in a San., romancing with another T.B. in the same San. But romancing with a soldier was a different matter altogether. It could have disastrous consequences.

When Irene wandered in one evening from a walk she shouldn't have been taking she had a quick wash, got undressed and went to bed without saying much to the other girls. Then she started putting her hair in curlers. Most of the girls spent a long time every night putting their hair in curlers. If they were going to die they were determined to die prettily.

Irene's silence worried them. They were used to her coming in tired but happy, and ready to tell them everything that had happened to her while she was out – or almost everything. There were things they had to press her to tell, and things she refused to tell however much they pressed, but she had never before come in without giving them something to share with her. At last one of them could bear her silence no longer.

'Is there anything the matter?' she called out

anxiously. Irene twirled a curl round her finger and peered at herself in a small mirror. Her flushed cheeks and bright eyes were worth peering at.

'I'm going home,' she said, putting the mirror down on the bed. The girls dropped their curlers and stared at her.

'But you can't,' said one of them when she had got enough breath back from the shock. 'You're only officially on Grade Two walks, you'll be in for ages yet.' Irene dipped her fingers in the glass of water on her locker and moistened a strand of hair.

'I don't care,' she said, twirling another curl. 'George has asked me to marry him and I've said I will, and nobody's going to stop me.' George was a soldier she had been seeing a lot of since he came to the gun site in the field. She had upgraded her walks so much that she had almost forgotten what her official grading was. The other patients had done some extremely dangerous cover-up work for her while she was defying authority. They were shocked at the unexpected turn their friendly collaboration had taken.

'But what will the doctor say?' they asked, knowing quite well what he would say. Irene arranged her lacy sleeping cap round her curlers then settled herself down in bed.

'I don't care what he says. I'm still going home,' she said. Then she shut her eyes to make the girls think she was asleep.

When the doctor did his round the next day Irene told him she was taking her own discharge to go out and marry her soldier. He told her not to talk such nonsense. She told him to mind his manners when he was talking to her. He pleaded; she was adamant. When he started to compromise she listened.

'Stay for another two months,' he begged her. 'I'll put you on longer walks then you might be ready to go out and go to your local clinic for check-ups.' He didn't know that she had already put herself on longer walks. When she still argued he brought out his ace.

'Think of George,' he said. She thought of George and finally decided that maybe two months was a small price to pay for a lifetime of happiness with him. George was a bit cross and said why not now while he was still there? Nobody knew where he might be in two months' time. But Irene soon calmed him down.

The girls asked their mothers to bring in materials. They stitched furiously all day and well into the night making clothes for Irene to look beautiful in when she walked down the aisle with George.

It was shortly after the last rosebud had been stitched into place on the veil that George was drafted somewhere a long way away and got killed by a German who was perhaps planning to get married himself on his next leave.

Irene wrapped up the silks and satin and told her mother to give them to anybody who needed a wedding outfit in a hurry. She didn't bother the doctor again about letting her go home. He wouldn't have, anyway. The longer walks had done her no good at all. She was in for a very long time.

As well as raising false hopes in girls with T.B. the soldiers had other uses. They were of inestimable value to us. Whenever they saw us taking the path across the field to the town they waved their bayonets at us and demanded to know whether we were friend or enemy. Usually, by the time we had advanced to be recognized, we were friends, though how close the friendship became depended on how short of friends we were at that particular time. The town was full of such imper-manent relationships. The cafés, cinemas and milk bars grew rich on them. There was tremendous rivalry between the soldiers from the fields and the airmen from the R.A.F. camp. But it was to the soldiers we turned when we came in late at night. And ironically, when we came in late because an airman had kept us out late. The soldiers knew all the rules we were supposed to keep and plenty of ways of breaking them without us getting caught.

'Will you be in late?' they asked, when their bayonets were safely back in the proper places. 'We will if we miss the last bus,' we promised them kindly. Missing the last bus was easy. Catching it was desperately hard. It either didn't run at all or it ran a long time before the big picture ended. Catching it meant us leaving the cinema before the villain was finally unmasked, while the heroine was beautifully breathing her last on a studio couch, or when the hero was in the throes of declaring his intentions, preferably down on one knee.

If we let the bus go and saw the end of the film we were faced with the long trek back to the hospital. However fast we ran the last few yards there were times when we fell by the wayside and arrived panting at the lodge gates long enough after ten to rouse the lodgeman's interest. This was where the soldiers came in useful. They could get us through the gates and into our bedroom windows with all the precision of a military manoeuvre. We were greatly indebted to them for their endeavours on our behalf. Even Davies had occasionally to solicit their aid, though it was a long time before she abandoned her principles enough to do so. The turning point for her came the night she was caught creeping up the drive with her shoes in her hand after a perfectly respectable evening spent down in the church hall knitting comforts for the troops. The sister flashed her torch for a split second on to Davies's face then in a voice of ice asked her where she intended telling the Matron she had been. Poor Davies didn't know. Telling her she had been knitting was too true ever to be believed. The excuse she invented had a far more wicked ring about it. After that if Davies thought she might be late she did the same as the rest of us did, and relied on the soldiers to get her in. But with one proviso. She made it clear that they would get no reward for helping her. This they respected. They saw in Davies the faithful sweetheart they hoped would be waiting for them when they got home. That they weren't too faithful themselves didn't strike them as important. They were men. Men were different.

The rewards they demanded varied with varying circumstances. Often they held us at ransom before they would lift a finger to help. If the ransom was too high and we haggled they either accepted a smaller due or left us to get ourselves in. Sometimes they got us over the sill first then dangled from the sandbags while they negotiated terms.

'Come to the pictures with us next week,' they begged, looking very silly with their noses pressed to the window. And we, safely in, would ungratefully spurn the offer.

'Sorry, I can't. I'm going with an airman next week.' This made the soldiers very angry, especially after all the trouble they'd gone to to get us in.

'Bloody pansies,' they said of the airmen. 'Never mind: you'll see, when this war really starts, it'll be us as will win it, not them blue-eyed boys down at the R.A.F. camp.' And off they would go, hissing angrily that it would be the last time they helped us over the window ledge. But the next time we needed them they were there, ready and willing to try again.

Later, when the war raged in the skies, we didn't

remind them of the things they had once said about the airmen. After all, they also were winning the war for us, and doing their best to keep the blue-eyed boys from being killed.

After Dunkirk we sent out more of the T.B. patients to make room for the men who didn't have T.B. Some of the lucky ones didn't have anything too awful at all, except their memories. They fell off the backs of lorries looking wet, sick and happy. There was plenty for them to be happy about. It was the ones they left behind who were unhappy.

They told us stories we found hard to believe. How was it possible for a man to come from France to England on a boat that had never been further than a trip round the lighthouse?

They told us stories of endurance and survival, of tremendous bravery and craven cowardice.

The ones who were wet, sick, and happy were dried out, given medicines to settle their stomachs and sent down to the R.A.F. camp to be kitted out, ready to go back for more, but not to Dunkirk. They quickly lost the first fine, careless rapture of survival.

Those who were brought in on stretchers were cleaned up and put to bed, cleaned up and taken to the theatre, or cleaned up and transferred to the mortuary.

When the visitors started coming and found their men in bed and not in the mortuary they were happy, until they saw the things that had been done to them on the beach and in our theatre. Then, though we worked hard at telling them their men were lucky to be alive, they still mourned over missing limbs and bandaged eyes. We soon discovered that the visitors suffered as much as the sufferers and were often the last to recover from the pain. Not having been at Dunkirk the picture the name conjured up was too terrible to think about. The glory only came afterwards.

The women walked up from the town offering food and beds for the visitors. They brought with them the results of the knitting orgies that had kept Davies out late at night. They unwrapped scarves that would have wrapped a mummy. They produced socks for giants and pullovers for pygmies. They carried baskets of hard-to-get fruit and dozens of impossible-to-buy eggs. And every mother treated every boy as if he was her own son, and every wife treated every man as she would have wanted her man to be treated had he been lying in a hospital a long way from home. Some already had sons and husbands a long way away from home. In prison camps. They looked at the men with bandaged eyes and wondered which was worse, that or the prison camp.

The war started getting into its stride after Dunkirk. The sirens sounded more often and were less often false alarms. Planes approached, roared overhead for a tense few seconds and roared off again, or they approached and were followed by a cacophony of sound from the gun site. We were still not experienced enough to know whether the plane was one of 'theirs' or one of 'ours'. When the war was over somebody tried to tell us that it was all in the mind, that 'theirs' and 'ours' were indistinguishable in sound. But we knew better. We were soon learning to look up when it was one of theirs and praying for one of ours to come and intercept it before it could do any damage.

But whether it was one of theirs or one of ours that plummeted down from the sky the crews died just as painfully, and often in our beds.

We were quickly learning to live with war. At night the searchlights gave more light than we had seen since the blackout began. We used it to light our way to the shelters with the patients who could walk there. We became very proficient at moving them quickly when the sirens went. We were equally proficient at talking those who couldn't walk into believing that they would be safe where they were; that the barricades were strong enough to keep them from harm. Some believed us, others didn't.

We almost grew fond of the guns in the field. While they banged away the enemy planes disappeared faster, so bang went the guns and hooray said everybody. Everybody except Charlie. Charlie didn't like the guns, they frightened him to death one day.

Charlie had been at Dunkirk. He didn't go to the theatre or to the mortuary when he got back, he simply went out of his mind. He was one of the last to get a lift home from France and while he was waiting and praying the guns fired incessantly, not to protect him but to kill him. After that Charlie had no faith in guns. It was no use telling him that the ones in the field were different, he was just as terrified of them as he'd been of the ones on the beach. While he was screaming his terror it took several of us to make sure that he wasn't doing anything that would stop the noise of the guns permanently for him. One day it all got too much for him and he fought us off while he did terrible things with an open razor he'd managed to steal from another patient's locker.

But despite things like Charlie happening life went on. We did fire drill, stirrup pump drill and evacuation drill. The stirrup pump drill wasn't always the serious exercise it was meant to be. The first time I saw Davies in her tin hat pumping away at a stirrup pump I almost fell into a fire bucket laughing. I didn't laugh so much when they told me I had to hold the end of the hose as near to a possible incendiary bomb as I could get it. The thought of what an incendiary bomb could do to me made me wish I was on the pumps like Davies, or even rushing backwards and forwards with the water.

And through it all there were still the little things to get upset about. The fact that there was so much happening around us didn't stop us from complaining bitterly about the food we got. However much we might have grumbled in peacetime about kippers for breakfast we found ourselves yearning for them passionately when we were faced with deep-fried fish paste sandwiches instead. We hated deep-fried sandwiches with whatever filling they had, but the fish paste was by far the worst. A scraping of fish paste on two slices of bread, coated with a watery batter and fried did nothing to tempt our appetites when we had been up half the night listening to the guns.

Neither did we care much for the hard cod's roe that was put in front of us regularly at suppertime, nor the branny stuff that was a substitute for sugar. It was a substitute for a lot of things. We threw it on stewed fruit to make the fruit less acid, we threw it into soup to make the soup less like cabbage water. Whatever we threw it on benefited little from the addition. All it did was make everything taste the same. When we did our complaining loudly enough for the housekeeping sister to hear she looked at us as if we were quislings or fifth columnists.

'Stop moaning and eat,' she said. 'Bran's roughage and cod's roes are vitamins. So eat them and think yourselves lucky you're eating at all, what with the U-boats and mines that are sinking our ships and drowning our merchant seamen.' We ate, but we avoided the deep-fried fish paste sandwiches as much as our hungry stomachs would let us.

The war was going on at my home as well. I got a

letter from my mother. 'Hope this finds you well,' it said. 'We are fine and the evacuees is fine but you remember that boy down the road you used to go on the school bus with? Well, he was took away last week. They said he was a blackshirt, whatever that might mean. Goodbye for now. Keep smilling.' The boy down the road had been a fanatical follower of Oswald Mosley for a long time. His mother, a proud and gentle woman, admired her son for his loyalty to his allegiances. Others condemned him for it. I kept an open mind, remembering the times he had done my homework for me at the back of the school bus. I was in no position to judge, having no clear idea about what I was judging.

Days went by and the nights passed. Things had just begun to fall into some sort of pattern when a gardener found a small bomb lodged between two branches of an apple tree. This changed the pattern completely.

Chapter Ten

Davies and I had gone to the pictures the afternoon the gardener stumbled upon the bomb in the apple tree. Luckily he didn't exactly stumble upon it, he just looked into the tree and there it was. Rumour had it that he was still shaking with fear long after he had finished telling everybody how fearless he'd been. But nobody was hard on him for that. Looking up into an apple tree and seeing a bomb was enough to shatter anyone's nerves.

Davies and I usually went to the pictures if we were off together on our half-days, and could afford it. Going in the afternoon was considerably cheaper than going in the evening. The audience was usually made up of old age pensioners as destitute as we were and one or two courting couples who hadn't gone there to watch the film.

The cinema we patronized was very basic. There was no organ to fill the intervals and technical hitches with melodic strains, and the interior had not been decorated since some of the old age pensioners were still courting couples. There were two other cinemas in the town but they were gilded and curtained beyond our pockets.

Though I was happy to accept an invitation to the pictures from a soldier or an airman whenever I got the chance I was just as happy to go with Davies if she wanted me to. Her dreams of seeing more of Archibald when we came nearer to London had not materialized. Whatever he was doing for his country took up a great deal of his time and when he did manage to see her the visit was too fleeting to do more than unsettle her for days after. The letters he wrote often came from a long way away and were so heavily scrawled across with blue pencil that she had to read more between the lines than she could have possibly read on them. She was still evasive when I asked her what he was doing. It was hard to tell whether she knew or not.

I realized that wearing his ring yet not having him available put Davies in a difficult position. Without a ring to cramp my life-style I was free to take up the offer of a milk shake, a bun and a cup of tea, or even a seat in the back row of the pictures. But Davies was not. She was committed to solitary walks and visits to the church hall where the women did their knitting and raised funds to buy Spitfires and Hurricanes. No self-respecting girl like Davies would have gone to the pictures alone or to a milk bar for an ice-cream soda. She was dependent on me for such shared delights.

We had smoked our way through several cigarettes

when the passionate love scene we were watching flickered and died. Several of the old age pensioners started stamping their feet and doing a slow handclap. Even the courting couples stopped whatever they were doing and joined in the booing. Things had just started to get out of control when the lights went up and the manager walked in front of the safety curtain. A spot light was focused on him and he raised his hand commandingly. Though it was the middle of the afternoon he was resplendent in evening dress. Its magnificence was wasted on the audience. It was also out of keeping with the shabbiness of the decor.

'Ladies and gentlemen,' he said in a loud voice. 'I have a message which I will proceed to read out if you will kindly keep quiet and let me read it.' We were shamed to instant silence and he read the message. 'Will all personnel from the sanatorium kindly leave the building at once. There is an emergency and they are needed back there at once.' He walked off the stage and the love scene sprang to life again. Davies looked at me through the tobacco haze that curled round our heads. 'That's us,' she said. We got up and walked down the row making everybody stand to let us pass. I trod on a few painful corns on the way.

On the road outside the cinema stood an old taxi-cab. As we left the cinema the driver rushed across to us with an anxious look on his face. 'Are you personnel from the hospital?' he asked. When we said we were he opened the cab door. 'You'd better get in quick,' he said urgently. 'You're wanted back as fast as I can get you there.' We got into the cab.

'What's happening?' asked Davies. The driver slammed the door and walked round to his own side. 'There's a bomb,' he said, getting in. Davies and I looked at each other in horror. 'Where is it?' she said. 'It's in a tree or something,' replied the driver. 'It hasn't gone off but it could if it shifted itself.' He closed the partition between us and him and we raced along the roads like a fire engine. The awful thought of what could happen if the bomb went off kept Davies and me silent until we reached the hospital.

The lodge gates were open when we got there and the taxi drove straight through and came to a screeching halt at the main entrance. Several other vehicles were standing there including some decrepit-looking old ambulances, a couple of buses and a few private cars. The driver threw himself out of his seat and rushed round to open the door for us. 'You'd better get yourselves in there fast,' he said, looking fearfully round him as if he expected to see the bomb hanging in mid-air somewhere. He got into the taxi and drove off.

'What shall we do about uniform?' I said to Davies, looking at our summer dresses and light stockings. 'We'd better go in first and see what's happening,' she said, 'then we can go across and change if we have to.' I glanced at her face. It was pale but apart from that she showed none of the fear I knew she felt. I hoped I was behaving as well as she was. We had been trained not to panic but we had never had a bomb to panic over before. Especially a bomb that could go off if it shifted itself. We walked up the steps and into the entrance hall.

In the hall there was a surge of people rushing about in all directions. Some were running. A sister hurried towards us with a pile of ambulance blankets in her arms. When she saw us she skidded to a stop, almost dropping the blankets in the skid. She looked hot and anxious.

'Hurry up, Nurses, and report to the Female block,' she cried breathlessly. 'There's a bomb in the apple tree outside the window and we have to evacuate the patients before anything terrible happens.' We also started to run.

When we got to the Female block a sister met us in the main corridor. She steered me one way and pushed Davies the other. 'Get yourselves into the wards at once,' she shouted. 'You'll have to help the juniors with the bedpan round then start getting the patients ready to be moved.'

'But, Sister,' I said, risking her anger, 'I thought there was a bomb just outside the window.' The thought of doing a bedpan round with a bomb waiting to go off outside the window struck me as being a bit reckless. The sister paused for a moment in flight.

'There is a bomb,' she said. 'And we must get the women away as soon as possible but they are all frightened to death and they are all gasping for a bedpan. If we don't give them one they'll be very uncomfortable on the journey. Especially if we're going a long way away.' I could see the sense in what she said. She grabbed a pile of pillows from a table and started off again. I went into the ward.

The nurses were passing the bedpans round with the smoothness of a conveyor belt. They looked a bit surprised when they saw me go into the sluice in my summer dress. I took some pans and joined the conveyor belt. The patients were sitting silently waiting for the bedpans. They were showing no sign of panic. Only their silence gave any indication of the strain they were feeling. In the sluice I managed to get some information.

'What exactly happened?' I asked as we washed and scoured. A junior turned to me eagerly. Nothing as exciting as this had ever happened to her and any fears she might have had were temporarily forgotten in the drama of the moment.

'The gardener found a bomb in the tree, it's caught up in a branch and it only needs a bit of wind to shift it.' I thought of the women sitting on their bedpans and prayed that there would be no wind.

'What are we supposed to be doing when they've had their bedpans?' I asked a third-year nurse who came into the sluice. She was not carried away by it all as the junior had been. She had a pinched look of fear in her face and her voice was sharp with worry.

'We're moving out,' she said. 'There are buses and ambulances coming to fetch us, then the bomb disposal men will come and defuse the bomb.'

'Have you any idea where we're going?' I asked her. She shook her head wearily. 'Nobody seems to know. Even Sister doesn't know. She keeps ringing round and asking people but nobody's told her anything.'

We still didn't know when the last bedpan had been given and the patients were ready in their dressing gowns and blankets to be loaded into the vehicles. As we wheeled those who couldn't walk we trod lightly. The fear of dislodging the bomb had mounted as time passed. There were one or two last-minute hitches before we were on our way.

'Nurse!' shouted a woman from one of the ambulances.

'What do you want?'

'It's me beads. I can't find them anywhere. They must still be in me locker.'

'Then they'll have to stay there, won't they? If you think I'm going back to get killed for the sake of a string of beads you've got another think coming.'

'But they're me rosary beads, Nurse. They're the only ones I've got.'

'Oh, all right then, but why you didn't make sure

you'd packed them I don't know.' And back went some-body, stepping warily lest they should be the one to rock the bomb. We needn't have worried. It stayed where it was until it saw the disposal men coming then it went off just to spite them. No one was hurt but there was enough damage done to keep us away for a long time.

We were just sitting back, thankful to be away, when somebody had another thought. 'What about us?' said a nurse. We looked at her.

'What are we going to wear?' she asked. Nobody had thought of that. Everybody had been so concerned with getting the patients away that we had been forgotten. It was another half an hour before we were finally on the road.

The ambulance I was in had four stretchers and several sitting patients crowded almost on top of each other. The journey would have been bad enough even if the ambulance had been in better condition. It was a rattling decrepit thing with scarcely the strength to keep one wheel moving in front of the other. Somewhere within its depths terrible things were happening all the time. It creaked and groaned, jolted and jerked, and came to sudden stops, throwing us into each other's arms and on to the stretcher cases. It was soon apparent that wherever we were going would be too far away for any of us. Tempers were already frayed with the strain of knowing about the bomb and the rocky ride we were having did nothing to improve them.

'Where are we going?' I asked the driver's mate when the ambulance stopped for yet another five or ten minutes while they looked for whatever had stopped it. The man gave me a dirty look. The journey was as hard for him as it was for us. 'We're going somewhere in the country,' he said impatiently.

'Which country?' I asked, putting a lot of sarcasm into the question.

'This bloody country, of course,' he replied, slamming the door furiously.

'Bad-tempered devil,' said a patient bad-temperedly.

We trundled along slowly, stopping and starting when things got too much for the poor old engine. It was almost dark when we finally drew up outside a pair of heavy iron gates encrusted with a gilded coat of arms. An old man came slowly out of the tiny lodge cottage and opened the gates. We proceeded like creaking royalty up the mile-long drive. At the end of it the man I had upset with my sarcasm flung open the ambulance doors.

'We're here,' he grunted.

'Thank God for that,' I said, massaging my tender bottom. The sitting patients, stiff and sore with sitting, got up and stretched themselves while I helped them down the steps. We left the stretcher cases until the men got round to dealing with them.

Through the shadowy end of summer light we could make out the shape of a large mansion with steps leading up to a massive front door.

'It's a bloody castle,' said one of the women, peering through the dimness. 'God knows where we are but wherever we are it don't look civilized to me.' Civilized to her meant plenty of bustle and people on the streets. Here there was neither. Maybe if we had listened more closely we would have heard the screech of an owl or the barking of a fox in the distance but none of us had any desire to hang about listening for such things. Least of all me.

'Come on,' I said briskly, 'let's get inside, it's chilly out here and you must all be dying for something to eat.' I was, so I guessed they were. We opened the doors and went inside, carefully closing the doors after us because of the blackout. The moment we were inside I knew that however hungry we were there would be no food for a long time. The great hall we were in was a milling scene of total chaos. Every inch of floor space was filled with stretchers and every inch of sitting space was already being sat on. The four more stretchers out of our ambulance added further to the confusion.

Davies had got there before me. Her ambulance had been in better shape. She looked very tired. Everybody looked very tired. I picked my way through the stretchers and went across to her.

'What's happening?' I asked her. She shook her head dejectedly.

'Nobody seems to know,' she said. 'I've been here nearly an hour and they're still trying to sort out where to put us all.'

I looked round.

'It's a bit baronial isn't it?' I said. It was indeed. The walls and floor were golden with age and loving care. The wood gleamed under the light of a massive chandelier that would have killed us as surely as a bomb if it became detached from its moorings. Standing about in corners were knights in shining armour, their lowered visors shutting out the common herd that was invading their privacy. Graceful women in white marble raised beckoning fingers and gazed beseechingly up to invisible suitors. A great staircase rose in sweeping curves to an upper landing. The curves were not designed to provide easy access for stretcher cases. When at last the time came for getting the patients upstairs things started to get more difficult than they were before. Bad language floated through the banisters as we and the men struggled with the stretchers.

'For God's sake watch what you're doing with your end of the thing.'

'I am watching what I'm doing. And don't you speak to me like that. Remember I'm a nurse, not a navvy.'

'I don't care if you're a bloody angel, all I'm asking you to do is to straighten your end up a bit.'

'I can't. If I straighten it up any more the patient will slip off altogether and go base over apex down the stairs.' This had the effect of alerting the patient to the danger she was in.

'Here, watch it. It's me on this trolley and don't you forget it. If you drop me I'll have the law on you.'

'Shut up and lie down.'

'Well, I'm only warning you.'

'Just shut up.' Voices rose, tempers rose, but in spite of it all nobody was dropped. We were almost as surprised as the patients were about that.

It was a long time before linen was found, beds made up and patients put into them. Not everybody was happy even then.

'Where's me pillow, Nurse?'

'It's under your head, where do you think it is?'

'No, it isn't, I haven't got one.'

'Of course you have.'

'No, I haven't.'

'Yes, you have.' Mutter mutter, grumble grumble. We were tired, they were tired and we were all at the end of our tethers. There was much still to be done. Being tired had to wait. The tethers had to be lengthened.

When all the patients were in bed, still muttering and grumbling about something, it was time for us to start looking for things to feed them with. We rummaged through boxes and dived into containers.

'I can only find tinned things,' said a voice from the depths of a tea chest.

'Then they'll have to have tinned things, won't they?' said somebody else deep inside a crate.

'And who, may I ask, is supposed to give out the suppers?' asked somebody, belligerently waving a tin opener around. 'There isn't a domestic in the place.'

There wasn't a domestic in the place because none had come with us. They were being sent on later after all the accommodation problems had been solved. We explained all this to the belligerent one. The explanation did nothing to appease her.

'Well, I think it's a disgrace,' she said. 'Why should we be expected to feed the patients when there are no domestics to feed them with?' We tried to get a little fun out of the idea of feeding patients with domestics but the joke fell flat and the nurse with the tin opener went off in a huff, taking it with her. We had to chase after her to retrieve it.

We gave the patients corned beef and bread and marge for their supper, keeping a little of the corned beef back for our own meal. There was no sugar to put in their tea, as somebody had forgotten to pack it. Luckily the war had reduced most people's sugar intake so there were fewer grumbles than there might have been.

When the patients had been fed and could be left on their own for a while we went into the dining-room and ate our corned beef. The dining-room was totally unsuitable for a meal of corned beef and bread and marge. It would have lent itself more happily to things like venison and sucking pig, with shrieking serving wenches hotly pursued by roistering, bottom-pinching knaves. From huge canvases on the walls sad eyes looked down at our meagre diet, remembering happier times.

After supper we set about looking for things that people had forgotten to send or that were quite impossible to find wherever they had been stowed.

'There aren't any hot-water bottles,' screeched someone from inside a cupboard.

'We won't need hot-water bottles,' said somebody else. 'We only give them hot-water bottles if they are outside in the chalets or on the verandahs. They're all inside here so they wouldn't be allowed a hot-water bottle.' She was right. The rules about the giving of hot-water bottles were inflexible. Though the patients' breath might freeze solid on the windowpane they got no hot-water bottles if they were within four walls. During the most untypical heat wave the patients sweltering outside in chalets were dutifully presented with a rubber bag of boiling water. Routine was a religion that had to be strictly observed.

'There isn't any porridge,' came another anguished cry. 'What do we give them for breakfast?' If there was no porridge we gave them something else, it sounded such a simple solution to an insoluble problem. But it wasn't so simple. Since the beginning of time hospital patients had had a bowl of porridge put in front of them to eat or leave as it pleased them. Mostly they left it. But for there suddenly to be no porridge for them to leave was another major catastrophe reflecting all the other catastrophes that had happened that day.

We got through the evening routine as best we could, with a scarcity of many essentials and a total lack of others, and after it was all done and the patients were settled, hopefully to sleep, we went round checking the blackout and getting ourselves better acquainted with our new surroundings. All the time we were being confused with little corridors that led nowhere and others that darkly concealed places vital to our needs. We hammered on doors that didn't open and fell down steps leading from those that did. Things that moved sent us gasping to cower near walls and things that fell with a crash in the distance had us reaching for tin hats.

When a terrible scream rang out from the direction of the lower hall we rushed to investigate, dreading what we might find. We found a little Irish nurse standing transfixed in front of one of the suits of armour. When she saw us she crossed herself devoutly and screamed again.

'Jesus, Mary and Joseph,' she yelled, crossing herself again. 'The bloody thing moved!' We looked at the shining knight. If he had moved he showed no signs of action now.

'It can't have moved,' we told her scornfully. 'It's been dead for centuries.' The thought of it being dead for centuries set the junior off again. 'I want to go back where we came from,' she moaned. 'I don't like it here.' Neither did any of us at that particular moment. We led her to the kitchen and told her to get on with doing the bread and marge for breakfast. With her trembling and shaking hands she sliced her fingers as much as she sliced the bread. The Holy Family had a busy time that night rushing to the kitchen every time she appealed to Them.

After we had done a round of all the long rooms that had been converted into wards and done anything anybody asked us to do for them we assembled again in the great hall to get our instructions from the senior sister who had come with us to deputize for the Matron. She looked as weary as we were. She looked round at us and sighed deeply. 'That's been a terrible time for you, I know,' she said gratefully. 'But I'm afraid there's more to come.' It wasn't possible, we thought. Nothing could be worse than the past hours. It could.

'There are not enough beds for us all,' said the sister, casting gloom so thick you could feel it in the air. 'Some of you will have to sleep in here and of course some of you will have to do night duty.' We had forgotten about night duty. The events of the evening had robbed us of all sense of time and order. We thought about night duty. There was no joy in the thought.

'How shall we keep awake?' said Davies who was standing next to me. I told her I didn't know but I was already asleep on my feet and doing night duty would kill me, I was sure. 'And me,' she said.

'How will we keep awake?' said Davies boldly to the

sister. The sister glanced at her sharply. 'You will do your duty, Nurse, I hope, in the way you have been trained to do it.' 'Yes, Sister,' said Davies. Then I astonished even myself. I had a brilliant idea.

'Please, Sister, couldn't we take it in turns to do night duty?' I asked, amazed at my own daring. 'We could do it in dog watches like sailors do.' I stood back expecting applause. There was none but there was a look of relief on the sister's face. Encouraged, I went on. 'We could do three hours at a time then come down for a rest.' And so we did, and hated every minute of it.

I was in the middle of a dream about Lord Haw-Haw hiding inside one of the suits of armour with the Irish nurse threatening to kill him with a slice of bread and marge when somebody woke me up. I leapt out of the chair expecting to see Lord Haw-Haw standing there but it was the nurse I was scheduled to relieve who was standing over me.

'Come on,' she hissed. 'These bloody dog watches were your idea so you'd better get up there and start doing some yourself.' I collected my senses and crammed a cap on my head. We had managed to bring enough uniform to see us through until fresh supplies arrived.

'What time is it?' I whispered.

'It's two o'clock and all's well. I'll come up when you call me and give you a hand with the morning work. Watch out for ghosts when you get up there,' she said, filling me with terror. I crept up the stairs struggling to keep my eyes open.

When I had gone round the ward I sat at a table and fought to stay awake. I also tried desperately not to be afraid. Since the beginning of my training night duty had filled me with strange fears. Over the years I had conquered most of the fears but that first night in our new hospital brought them all back to me. Plus a great many more. Shapes and shadows loomed in unexpected places, setting my nerves on edge. The faintest scamper from behind wainscoting or the slightest creak from anywhere almost stopped my breath. I sat until I could sit no longer then I got up and walked between the beds. One of the women lifted up her head and spoke to me.

'Are you all right, Nurse?' she whispered softly. I felt ashamed that she should be asking me when it was I who should have been asking her.

'Yes, I'm all right, thank you,' I said, trying to make myself believe it. 'Why aren't you asleep?' I stood beside the bed wishing from the bottom of my heart that I was in it.

'I don't know,' she whispered. 'I got off at first then something woke me. It's the bed I expect. It's rotten hard.' I sat down on the bed and took her hand in mine. It was hot and dry. I felt her pulse and it was racing. I was sorry I had envied her her bed. However tired I was I had two good lungs and a pulse that didn't race except in special circumstances. Tiredness was temporary, T.B. often wasn't.

'It's funny us being here, isn't it?' said the woman softly. 'How long do you think we'll be here?' I didn't know but I gave some sort of answer. She was quiet for a moment then she spoke again. 'It's a lot further away from London than the other place was, isn't it? Will our visitors be able to get here?' I assured her they would. Despite the time we had taken to get there the place wasn't any further away from London, it was just in a different direction.

I gave her back her hand and stood up. 'I'll go and make you a hot drink,' I said. 'It will send you back to sleep.' I went to the kitchen and warmed some milk. When I got back to the ward with it the woman was already asleep so I went back to the kitchen and drank it myself. She had missed nothing – it was horrible.

It was shortly after I had drunk the milk that I almost died of fright. And caused the patients almost to die of fright at the same time.

The moment anybody was admitted to the T.B. wards with a tubercular spine they were put into a plaster cast in order to immobilize the spine. The casts were made of plaster of Paris and exactly fitted the patient's shape. Spares were made and stored in a cupboard in a bathroom. Or they were stored in a bathroom in normal circumstances. But the circumstances that night were far from normal. I walked into a lavatory, switched on the light and turned round. Behind the door, casually leaning against the wall, was a figure, all in white. Not waiting long enough to discover that the figure was a plaster cast that somebody had put there until a more suitable place was found for it I gave a tremendous scream and rushed out of the lavatory.

We started the morning work much earlier that day than we usually did. There seemed no point in not doing so when all the patients were awake and all the nurses had rushed upstairs to find out why I was screaming. I was in very serious trouble with the sister-in-charge and very unpopular for a long time with the other nurses. None of them would admit that they might have reacted just as uncontrollably if they had walked into a lavatory and found a ghost leaning against the wall.

When we heard the dawn chorus we went to the end of the ward and drew aside the blackout curtains. All around us were dark pine forests. We could smell their scent from where we stood. The women hated them. A plane tree standing in the middle of a London square they didn't mind, but rows upon rows of menacing trees were not at all to their liking. They were no more enthusiastic about the joys of country life than their children had been when they saw their first cow.

The morning work was as tedious as the evening's had been. Being even more tired we found it harder to cope with. We were used to the soft life – having things that we needed in the place they were expected to be. Here nothing was where we could find it. We spent precious time substituting for this and searching frantically for that. The substitutions were not always successful.

'Whatever's that?' I asked a junior who was staggering from the kitchen with an enormous fish kettle. 'It's a fish kettle,' she replied, looking surprised that I didn't know. 'What are you doing with it?' I inquired curiously. 'I'm boiling the patients' eggs in it,' she said, buckling beneath the weight. 'But there's a hole in the bottom of it,' I said, indicating the hole. 'I know,' she said glumly. 'I just let the eggs boil dry and the bottom nearly fell out.' She staggered away before the bottom completely fell out. Her efforts were wasted. After the first egg was hammered open the rest were left beside the uneaten bread and marge. Having no porridge to complain about the women weren't to be placated with rock-solid eggs.

When somebody opened one of the french windows at the end of the ward to let in a bit of fresh air a red squirrel came in with the fresh air. He sat and stared boldly round at the intruders. One of the women noticed him and screamed almost as loudly as I had screamed in the lavatory earlier. 'What is it?' she said, shaking with fright. 'Somebody come quick and make it go away. It's got no right to be in here, the nasty dirty thing.' It was neither nasty nor dirty. It was a beautiful creature, soon to be banished by its dull grey cousins.

'Don't be daft,' said another woman, walking down the ward softly so as not to frighten the squirrel away. 'It's only a squirrel. He won't hurt you. He's just dropped in for breakfast.'

After that the squirrel dropped in every morning for his breakfast. He was never sent away empty. He put on more weight than the patients did.

Chapter Eleven

IF THE SQUIRREL put on more weight than was good for him while he was living on the fat of our ward we lost some of ours with the exercise we got from walking from our lodgings to the hospital. Accommodation in the mansion was limited and not nearly sufficient to meet the needs of the patients and personnel that had been thrust upon it. Consequently most of the staff-nurses and some of the sisters were farmed out to various lodges scattered round the estate. Davies and I were banished to a tiny cottage that was hidden among a dense patch of undergrowth and surrounded on all sides by trees.

Because of the nearness of the trees and the almost hysterical precautions that had been taken to protect the cottage from a highly unlikely all-out enemy attack there was hardly any light at all in the house. It was as dark by day as it was by night. Neither had it any of the luxuries we had grown accustomed to over the years. We were back to oil lamps and an evil-smelling privy at the bottom of the garden. And candles to light us to bed.

But if no light was allowed to get in none was allowed to escape. The blackout material was a fixture at the windows and any gleam from the oil lamp that attempted a getaway when a door was opened was too faint for the most alert air-raid warden to worry about. The low success rate of the lighting system was due to the glass chimney of the lamp being so smoked up with use that it reached less than a quarter of its potential.

The old lady who became our landlady had lived in the lodge since the day she was carried over the threshold by a lusty young gamekeeper on the estate. From all she told us he must have been as fertile as the eggs he was paid to protect. At the last count she gave us their family had numbered thirty, give or take a few miscarriages and false alarms. But since the old lady got the sum wrong every time she totted it up we quickly lost faith in her statistics.

We had listened at first with bated breath but later in acute boredom to the account of her many labours; each pang and pain made more graphic by the groans and grimaces with which she illustrated the story. If she confused the 'emmeridge' she had when her Sally was born with the caul that adhered when Willy arrived she would look at us apologetically. 'No, take it back, I tell a lie,' she would cry, then proceed to go through the entire gestation period again, arriving in the fullness of time at the moment when the infant was safely delivered into her care. Soon we were able to fill in her lapses of memory ourselves. 'No, love,' we would hastily remind her, 'it was Georgy not Johnny who gave you the prolapse.' And she, after casting around in her mind, would admit we were right and instead it had been Johnny who made her teeth fall out. She was perfectly aware that something fell out after she'd had her Johnny but she could never be sure if it was her teeth or her womb. It was varicose veins with Vincent.

Because of her great age she wasn't expected to put herself out too much for us, her duties being mainly to see that we came in at a respectable hour at night. 'Respectable' for her was nine o'clock but she unwillingly stretched it to ten if we pleaded hard enough. Whether we came in at nine or ten made little difference to the reception we got. By ten o'clock she was always in bed and sound asleep and we, being allowed no latch key, had to wake up all the wild life in the woods with our knocking. By the time the old woman had lit her candle, put on her shawl, shuffled into her slippers and spent several minutes being assured that it was indeed us and not a prowler come to do an old lady to death we had decided that nothing was worth the aggravation of staying out until ten o'clock at night.

But coming in at nine wasn't easy. By nine o'clock our landlady had begun the slow process of getting ready for bed and if she was in the scullery having a rinse, or in front of the fire halfway between corsets and nightdress, it could take just as long for her to consent to let us in.

She had made it clear when we were first foisted on her that we would have to fend for ourselves in the mornings. Fending for ourselves meant that most mornings we were too lazy to get up and make ourselves a cup of tea. We trailed through the wakening woods along damp bridle paths and into the mansion, often too late for breakfast and already weary from the walk.

The living-out arrangements were that we should eat our main meals at the mansion when we were on duty and any snacks we needed were to be taken at our lodgings. There were certain drawbacks to the arrangements. One of these was the state of the crockery we were expected to eat and drink from. Like the old woman the pots got a rinse rather than a proper wash and were grimy enough to put us off eating and drinking for ever. The other drawback was the dog.

The dog was very large. He took up most of the living-room. He was not a ferocious dog or even the least bit unfriendly. He was just an ordinary dog with a tail that wagged, knocking everything off tables and lashing at our legs. He was man's best friend. But he was more than a friend to the woman we lodged with. To her he was husband, child and father. He shared her hearth, her meals and her bed. Side by side they slept, keeping each other warm when the wind shook the small cottage. To say he was faithful to her would be an understatement. They had lived together so long that he was part of her and she of him. We understood their devotion and were happy about it. We were glad they had each other to turn to on the cold winter nights. What we were not happy about was the old lady's insistence that we share our snacks with the dog. Encouraged by her he stood beside our chairs while we ate, drooling at the mouth and following each bite from plate to lips, panting in ecstatic anticipation. Unless we gave in to his panting the old woman took it as a slight on her and her dog. She sulked with us and told the dog what nasty unfeeling things we were. In the end we were giving him all the tastiest morsels and most of the chunkiest chunks. This could leave us very hungry if we were relying on the snacks as main meals.

When we could bear it no longer we went to the sister-in-charge and asked her if we could be moved. She raised her eyebrows and accused us of making a lot of fuss about nothing. It was only after she had been to the cottage and seen for herself that we were permitted to pack our bags and go to one of the other lodges. Even there we had problems. But instead of being robbed of our food we were deprived of sleep.

The lodge was occupied by a young married couple. The man was another lusty gamekeeper who had only recently rushed his bride into the front door and up the stairs. They were still in the first flush of the honeymoon and until he got his call-up papers and went off to be killed we were kept awake late and wakened often during the night by a lot of heavy breathing and cries of ecstasy coming from the bridal chamber. Though the walls were thick the sounds were penetrating and from them we guessed that the new husband spent a lot of time chasing his beloved round the room. His beloved didn't seem to object and soon we grew tired of pressing our ears to the pillow to exclude the clucking and crowing and resigned ourselves to yet another disturbed night. I started listening enthralled, and even Davies wore a wistful look sometimes.

Near to the hospital but separated from it by a tree-lined walk was a garrison town packed to the smallest alley with soldiers. There were enough of them to go round all the local girls and plenty left over for any itinerant nurse who happened to want one. Most of the soldiers were bent – to a greater or lesser degree – on finding consolation for being torn from wives and sweethearts. The tree-lined walk offered every facility for an unattached young woman lucky enough to find an unattached young man among the crowds in the High Street. None but the most churlish soldier would expect the young woman to walk back from the pictures alone, especially if he had paid the ninepence to get her into the pictures. With the hospitality of the Forestry Commission there was every chance that the two of them would get better acquainted on the way through the woods.

Sadly, things didn't always go as they were expected to. Often the walk had only just got into its stride when the soldier dived into his inside pocket and brought out a photo of his young lady, dressed specially for the photo in her best peep-toe shoes and currently fashionable turban. When the picture had been oohed and aahed over it was firmly established that the walk through the trees was an act of gallantry only and not to be taken as a prelude to romance. Sometimes it was a wife or a fat bonny baby that shattered any hope there might have been for the future.

But even if there was no development from a Kodak Brownie camera to spoil things the hoped-for love story could still end unhappily. Just as the walks had begun to get interesting the soldier would deliver the bad news that he was shortly to be posted to a place too distant for him to keep in touch. There was often a slight discrepancy between the given details of the posting and the way it actually happened. Much anguish could result from the harrowing farewell scene that was played outside the lodge gate. Even more anguish could result when the dear departed was discovered in the town the following night with his arm wrapped tightly round another girl. The one to emerge from these confrontations the most happily was the dear departed himself. He had played the scene so often he could carry it off without batting an eyelid.

Another thing that could canker the love-in-bloom

faster than an attack of greenfly was a simple question like 'When are we going to get engaged?' Such pinning down could play havoc to the tender flowering thing that was but a shoot. There was nothing more certain to send a serviceman fleeing for his life than to be asked to state his intentions, particularly if he had no intentions to state. It was due to one of these unfortunate mishaps that I was walking alone through the woods the night I looked across in the direction of London and saw a dull red glow in the sky. I stood and watched, then, as the glow spread and got brighter, I raced all the way back to the mansion and burst into the sitting-room.

'Come outside,' I shouted, breathless with shock and running. 'London's burning.' The resident nurses who were sitting round the fire reading or listening to the wireless looked up irritably. Being non-resident I had no right in their sitting-room at all. They strongly resented the intrusion.

'For God's sake stop being so dramatic,' said one of them, laying down her book. 'What are you talking about?'

'It's London,' I gasped. 'It's burning. There's a huge red glow coming from there and you can see the flames shooting up.' Somebody got up and turned off the wireless.

'Come outside,' I begged desperately. 'You'll see for yourselves then.' At last they were impressed and we all rushed out of the front door. The glow in the sky had spread, and criss-crossed everywhere were the beams from a multitude of searchlights. We could see the flashes of light as the anti-aircraft guns went into action.

'My God, you were right,' said the nurse who had accused me of dramatics. 'It really is burning.' Nobody else said anything. There seemed nothing to say in the face of such terrible happenings. Then a sister came out of the front door. She wasted no time looking up to the skies. 'Get inside at once,' she said sternly. 'You'll all be needed on the wards when the patients from London find out what's going on there.' Most of us were not in uniform, some of the residents were even in their dressing gowns but we went to the wards without questioning the sister. It would need more than the few night-nurses on duty to cope with terror-stricken women when they started asking questions. It wasn't long before they were asking them.

'What's happening, Nurse?' they asked, jostling each other to get to the windows. Those who couldn't get up to look were even more fearful than those who could. Seeing things for themselves might have been easier for them than lying in bed conjuring up pictures. We spent the night thinking up ways of telling the women who came from dockland that it wasn't happening in the docks, and the women who came from wherever that it wasn't their homes that were being burnt to the ground. While we were telling our lies the thunder of wave after wave of fighter planes added to the confusion. None of us went to the shelters. Commonsense told us we should, but all of us felt the need to share some of the agony that London was suffering that night.

In the middle of it the young woman from the lodge where I lived came in, shaking with fear and dread. Her husband had volunteered to join the queue of fire engines that was winding its way through the lanes and to the city. He wasn't a fireman but he was a strong young man who could use his strength wherever it was needed.

The next morning Lily was very late coming in to work. Lily was one of the women who trudged up from the town to do the work of two or three domestics when they were released for more important jobs. She was hard-working and conscientious and had never been late for anything in her life. The sister was very angry when she saw Lily.

'Where do you think you've been?' she asked her. To everybody's surprise Lily burst into tears. This was as much out of character for her as being late for work. Her chirpiness had cheered us many times when we needed cheering. She was a joy to have around. We pushed her into a chair and made her a cup of tea. There had been so many cups of tea made on the ward that night that we had quite forgotten it was against the rules. Rules had suddenly become less important.

'I've been up all night,' said Lily laying her head on the kitchen table. We remembered then that we had all been up. We made yet more tea and drank it while Lily told us her story. After she had finished telling it we wished we had more to offer her than tea. Something like a medal, for instance.

She told us that throughout the night car-loads and lorry-loads of women and children had streamed into the town until the common was seething with them, the fields had room for no more and they were spilling over into people's gardens. Lily said that everybody in the town had made tea, cooked whatever meal they could manage to put together, and taken in the children who should have been sent to safety long ago instead of having to be bundled on to a lorry when it was almost too late.

Beds were made up on floors, in attics and even in baths. Not, Lily said, that many slept in them, except of course the children who were tired enough to sleep anywhere so long as a bomb didn't go off just as they were shutting their eyes. Lily finished her story then went into the ward to do the thousand and one things she was expected to do while there was a shortage of domestics. In between waxing and buffing the floors, sweeping and dusting, scrubbing and polishing she managed to take time off to comfort the patients and assure them that things were not as bad as they thought they were. Knowing as she did that things were far worse than they could ever have imagined it required considerable skill on Lily's part to make her assurances convincing.

When she had done all she was paid to do and a great deal more besides, she went to the sister and shuffled nervously in front of her.

'Please, Sister,' she said anxiously, 'would you mind if I went off a few minutes early today?' She was deeply ashamed at having to ask a favour so soon after she had disgraced herself by coming on duty late. The sister looked at her.

'Why?' she wanted to know.

'Please, Sister,' said Lily, 'I promised I'd go back to the rest centre when I'd finished here and cook some more meals for the refugees.' She shuffled her feet again.

'Oh, all right,' said the sister. 'I suppose if you promised you'd better go but mind you're not late again in the morning.'

'No, Sister,' said Lily and went. The sister stood for a moment watching her go. Then she turned to her own problems of trying to stop the patients taking their own discharge. This time it was harder than it had been before.

'You'll only get worse if you go out now. Then where will you be?'

'I'll be where I ought to be while this lot's happening.'

'But it will kill you going down to the shelters every night.'

'Maybe it will and maybe a bomb will but at least I'll die at home and not stuck here in the middle of nowhere.' There was no answer to that. The chances of a bomb killing them or their dying with T.B. were fairly even if they lived in London.

When the news started coming in we worked harder at sharing grief than we did at nursing tuberculosis. Visitors came when it wasn't visiting day. They brought tidings that could just be endured and tidings that nobody could bear to hear. But always there was Lily to make them more bearable.

'I've got a houseful now,' she told us soon after the first glow had appeared in the sky.

'A houseful of what?' we asked.

'Them evacuees, of course,' said Lily. We might have known. She told us they were not always the same evacuees. They came and went which made it harder on the washing what with having the sheets to change every time. The mangling and ironing took hours, she told us.

Some of the evacuees had rushed down from London in terror when a bomb fell on the street where they lived. Others arrived weary from fighting the fires the bombs had caused. The homeless came looking for shelter then went back, ashamed to be running away while friends and neighbours stayed behind watching everything falling in ruins around them.

A few men came down at night but left again in the morning to go to work. War or no war they had to eat and the children had to be fed; only by working could they get enough to eat. Sometimes they got back from work sooner than they expected to. It was no use staying when the place they worked was no more than a hole in the road and a heap of rubble.

When one family didn't come back at all Lily asked around. She was told that the family had decided to stay at home that night. They went to the shelter and in the morning the shelter wasn't there. All these things upset Lily very much but through it all she had an unshakeable faith in Mr Churchill. 'Good old Winnie,' she said when she saw pictures of him with a large cigar in his mouth peering down bomb craters. When he put out his call for blood, sweat and tears Lily cheered and unstintingly offered everything she had. She also gave unstintingly of herself.

After Bella's visitors came and told her that her children had been killed somewhere in the country where they had been evacuated to safety Bella wouldn't listen. Her mother sat with tears streaming down her face while she tried to make Bella look at the telegram that had been sent that morning. Bella had no intention of looking at the telegram. Seeing it down in black and white would have made it true and that was the last thing Bella wanted it to be. She wanted to go on believing that her children were on a farm doing things they had been forbidden to do, and not buried deep beneath the school that a German bomber had chosen for his target the night before.

It was Lily who finally made Bella face up to the fact that her children were dead. When neither Lily nor Bella could be found one afternoon we asked the few remaining patients if they knew where they were. They said they had seen the two of them going out through the door but none of them knew where. The sister did a bit of mumbling and grumbling because being a sister it was expected of her; then she put her trust in Lily and waited. Suppers were over and the medicines had been given out before they came back. Bella went straight to bed but we noticed she was crying a little instead of staring into space. When we asked Lily about it she seemed to take it for granted that helping to mend broken hearts was just another of the things Mr Churchill would have expected of her.

'How did you do it?' we asked her.

'I just took her into the woods where it was quiet and we sat under a tree and talked.'

'What did you talk about?' we asked.

'Oh, just things,' said Lily vaguely. 'I told her bits about my kids and the things they got up to when they was babies. Then she told me about her kids and the things they did. Then we had a laugh about how we'd belted them if they didn't do as they was told. Then we had a good cry and then we came back. Will she be all right now, Nurse?' It would take time but Bella would be all right – thanks to Lily and her powers of healing.

When the young Spanish girl in the bed in the corner learned that her parents wouldn't be coming to see her again she turned her face to the wall and stopped eating. This went on until we began to envisage a time when she would be going off to be with her parents again. Lily was desperate.

'That young Italian girl hasn't eaten nothing again today,' she kept telling us.

'She's Spanish,' we told her. Lily was surprised. They all looked alike to her, she said.

'Why don't you make her eat something?' she said, making it sound as if we were neglecting our duty.

'How can we make her eat if she won't?' we asked, a little crossly. We were as worried as Lily was.

'Maybe she don't like the food she gets,' she said, shoving a wartime rissole under our nose.

'And what's wrong with the food?' we asked, knowing only too well.

'Well,' said Lily. 'You must admit you don't like it much and you're English. Why don't you try her with something Spanish?'

'What sort of something Spanish?' Lily gave the problem a few minutes' thought. 'How about a bit of Spanish fly or something like that?' After we had carefully explained to Lily the various uses that Spanish fly was put to, none of them of a nutritional nature, she had another think. 'All right then, if Spanish fly's no good what about that young priest what comes in to see her?' For a moment we thought the young priest was to be sacrificed to provide the Spanish girl with nourishment. Lily was not amused when we questioned her about it.

'I meant tell him about her not eating,' she said with dignity.

'What do you expect the priest to do about it?' we asked her. She didn't know but the next time the priest came we told him the girl refused to eat. Lily kept butting in with her suggestion about a bit of something Spanish and the next day he came to the ward carrying a yard or two of flat dried fish and a bottle of olive oil. 'Give her this,' he said. 'She'll eat.' We sliced up the fish and marinated it in the oil then offered it to the girl. At first she wasn't interested in the offering but after Lily had had a little talk to her she sat up and started facing life again. She also ate the dried fish.

Lily had another moment of glory when Evelyn found a German airman standing on the drive with his parachute still harnessed to him. Evelyn was fifteen and had been blind since birth and tubercular almost as long. She had lived in a sanatorium for most of her life. Because of her blindness she had developed an inbuilt radar system that astonished everybody with its accuracy. We never ceased to marvel at it.

'How did you know it was us and not somebody else?' we asked her after every brilliant bit of identification she'd made. 'It's your huffs,' she said, making it sound as if we all had B.O. 'What are they?' we asked. Evelyn looked directly at us and gave us an indirect answer.

'They're just huffs,' she said. 'You've all got one and they're all different and I just know the difference.' That was as far as any of us ever got to understanding how her system worked.

Evelyn was a wanderer. She was never where she should have been. At medicine time she was in the kitchen helping with the washing-up and at mealtimes she had to be fetched from some part of the hospital grounds where she had gone off to have a chat with a gardener. She only chatted to the ones whose huffs she liked. Others she swept past and ignored. They foolishly thought this was the way of a blind girl. We could have told them the cut was deliberate. She was very selective with her friendships.

The gardener she liked best was old Jack. He was long past the age when he should have been working. He had been fetched back to replace a younger man who had gone off to join the Navy and would be dead while Jack was still pottering about among the roses and hydrangeas. It was when Evelyn thought she had found Jack that she was actually standing in the path of the German airman. We heard all about it when the excitement was over.

189

'Whatever happened?' we asked Evelyn.

'I was going down the path to find Jack,' she said.

'And she thought he was there in front of her,' broke in Lily.

'And he wasn't,' said Evelyn.

'It was this German with a parachute on,' explained Lily.

'And then I realized it wasn't Jack's huff',' said Evelyn, 'and I started screaming because I didn't know whose huff it was.'

'Then I heard her scream and I rushed out and there she was stuck right in front of this Jerry.' Lily looked at Evelyn proudly. 'He never knew she was blind, you see, because she was standing looking straight at him.'

They both got their pictures in the local papers though little was said about what had happened. Careless talk cost lives as everybody was constantly being warned but Lily made it her business to see that everybody knew the daring deed she and Evelyn had done between them.

The airman was very put out when he learned that he had been captured by a blind girl. It was a severe blow to his pride. The police said afterwards that he wasn't a bad sort of a chap, considering he was a German. Evelyn agreed with them. She said his huff was really quite nice. Except that she hadn't recognized it.

By this time the sirens were going night and day. Fighters went over, bombers went over, theirs and ours disturbed our nights and made the days full of incident. Everybody was starting to behave as if war was something they had lived with all their lives. Air-raid wardens and civil defence personnel who had complained at the boredom of it all began to long for a little of the boredom to return. Rumour spread and was denied, or was found to be true, with the truth even more terrible than the rumour had been. A bomb fell in a town not near enough to do us any damage but near enough to damage the lives of people we knew and friends we loved. The lives of everybody were being affected in some sort of way. Everybody had a story to tell. Visitors came down from London unless there had been a bomb en route to stop them. They sat at the bedside boasting about 'their' bomb. Their own special bomb. The one that had fallen on their house while they were in the shelters, on their street while they were somewhere else, the bomb that was just a little bit bigger than the bomb that had destroyed their mate's house in some other part of London. The bomb had begun to be spoken of with a little pride and even a little affection, unless it had cost too much in human suffering. Even then those who had managed to survive could still boast about their survival. There was a lot of interesting speculation made during visiting time. 'If the bloody thing had dropped a minute later' (or a minute earlier) 'I wouldn't be sitting here now talking to you.' 'If I'd been standing on that side of the street instead of where I was my name would have been on the one they dropped last night.' It was amazing the difference a moment of time or a fraction of an inch could make to a life.

We still had no bomb of our own to boast about. There had been a few stray incendiaries that pitted the lawns with brown patches and left the roofs and guttering not as safe as they were before. But until the day I was helping an exiled Rumanian doctor with a bit of minor surgery nothing spectacular had happened. He had just reached the point of no return in his examination of a patient when he looked over my shoulder and through a window. What he saw made his hand shake for a split second then he recovered himself and gave me a warning look. I took a quick glance through the window, lost my concentration for a moment then got it back before the patient noticed anything was wrong. Since there was nothing we could do to speed up the job we were doing we went on almost as if there were not more than a dozen incendiaries lighting up the lawn. The patient couldn't have done anything about it, anyway. She was lying on her side with a huge needle in her back. One false move and the needle would have slipped, wasting the precious spinal fluid the doctor was collecting for a specimen. She might not have lain so still if she had known what was going on outside the window. And there was plenty going on. Plenty that we only heard about after it was all over.

We stayed where we were for a long time, telling the patient that it was to her advantage to lie quietly until we moved her. Then we wheeled her to the ward where the other women were. Most of them were still standing at the windows watching the end of operation incendiary. It had all gone fairly smoothly, they told us. As in all operations there were one or two setbacks. The chain gang of nurses who were delegated to supply the sweating doctors with enough water to keep the pumps going had done a splendid job apart from one or two moments when they either collapsed under the strain or didn't get the shuttle movement right. The ones who were manipulating the hoses had a tendency to change direction midstream and instead of dowsing the flames almost drowned the passing water carriers. But by some miracle the incendiaries had all been made harmless by the time outside help arrived. Those who had helped to bring about the miracle talked of nothing else for days. They had just got back to ordinary conversation when the real bomb fell.

We were in the middle of giving out the dinners when the crash came.

'My God, we've been hit!' screamed a patient. 'No, we haven't,' said another. 'If we had been hit we wouldn't have heard the bang. They say you never hear the one that hits you.' None of us was too sure about the infallibility of the maxim. Somebody dived under the ward table, one or two of the patients threw themselves beneath the beds and others jammed themselves in the small linen cupboard. A nurse who had lived since the day war broke out in mortal dread of a bomb falling stood very still for a moment or two then walked calmly down the ward and threw herself across a patient who couldn't have moved an inch to avoid the large piece of masonry that threatened to fall from the ceiling down on to her bed.

When the sister had picked herself up from the floor where the blast had flung her she clapped her hands sharply. 'Come along, Nurses,' she called. 'We are still alive and there's work to be done.' We came out from wherever we had been hiding looking slightly ashamed of ourselves. We had not been hit. The bomb had fallen in the grounds sending the hens squawking and cackling with an early moult and the donkey that lived a quiet life in a corner of a field braying with astonishment.

We got the patients back into their beds after we had brushed the litter away and then made cups of strong tea for them and us. The tea ration was severely cut after that day.

When somebody asked where Evelyn was nobody knew. Lily went out to look for her and brought her back. She had heard the bang and the donkey braying. She had missed the great crater that appeared in the bridle path where she usually took a morning stroll. For a reason that she couldn't explain she had gone the other way round for a change. There must have been a huff about the bomb that she went out of her way to avoid. Even before it fell.

The mansion got a new look. Knights in armour lay on the floor in the great hall, badly dented where chunks of ceiling had fallen on them. Some had sustained more damage than they appeared to have done during the bloodiest combat in their youth. Marble statues stared up at us with cold and sightless eyes as inscrutable as the Mona Lisa and with fewer limbs left than the Venus de Milo could boast. Birds that had found their last resting places in the huge chimneys landed in sooty heaps in the fireplaces along with a lot of other interesting debris. Rafters hung crazily from roofs and slates lay about everywhere together with the glass they had shattered on their flight through the impregnable windows.

Faced with more than we could cope with we appealed to Lily and she raced down to the town and came back with as many evacuees as she could find to help sweep the floors and pick up knights. She was in her element as a works forewoman. She bullied and bellowed and showed us a side of her that we had never seen before. It was a side the evacuees hadn't seen either but they responded to it. It was good practice for those who would have clearing up of their own to do when they went back to their blitzed homes.

But despite our efforts and despite all the hard work

Lily and her gang did the mansion needed more care than we were able to give it to make it habitable again. Soon we were once more on the move. Back again to the main hospital.

Chapter Twelve

BECAUSE THE HOMECOMING journey had been arranged without the urgency of the outgoing one it was better organized, but there were still enough delays along the way to stretch it out even longer. This time the delays were less the fault of decrepit old ambulances and mainly caused by planes at the peak of their efficiency. Or they were at the peak of efficiency when they left base. Whether they reached their target at the same level was something that often needed to be decided almost immediately above us. It was this decision-making that had us lurking in the shelter of hedgerows when we should have been racing along at a heady twenty miles an hour on the main roads.

The battles in the sky were terrifying enough to make us tremble at the knees when the sirens wailed but fascinating enough to keep us at the windows watching until the All Clear sounded. We arrived at the hospital late but mercifully all in one piece.

It was still light enough when we got there for us to see that some changes had been made during our absence. The changes manifested themselves when we were halfway up the drive. Instead of the unhindered sweep of the gravel path past the sanatorium, away to the Administration block and beyond to the nurses' home, there was now what looked like a traffic island midway between the lot. When the ambulance I was in drew up outside the main entrance I scrambled out of it and looked at the innovation in amazement.

'Whatever is it?' asked a woman standing behind me.

'It's a sort of traffic island,' I said brightly, walking round to get a better view. The woman followed me round. 'Anybody can see it's a sort of traffic island,' she said scornfully. 'What I want to know is what it's doing stuck out here in the middle of the drive?' We continued to inspect the island.

Dead centre of it there was a signpost with three arms and black letters painted on the arms. I read the letters. The arm pointing towards the nurses' home had 'Nurses' Home' painted on it. This failed to excite me. I was well acquainted with the nurses' home and needed no signpost to tell me where it was. Neither did I have any doubts about the location of the Admin. block or the San. I could have found both with my eyes shut. The thing that had me and the woman looking at the signpost in wonder was the third arm. It pointed directly across to where the soldiers had been in occupation when we left. On it in bold black letters was printed 'Annexes – 1–10'. I read it several times trying to make some sense of it.

'What are them things?' asked the woman, looking at me expecting enlightenment. I had none for her. I was as ignorant as she was but I had no intention of telling her so.

'They must be some different sorts of soldiers,' I said briskly. The woman was not taken in.

'How can they be some sort of soldiers?' she asked. 'If they was some sort of soldiers they'd hardly put up a notice telling everybody where they was. Supposing an enemy came down the drive and saw some sort of soldiers on a signpost, he'd be across there like a shot with his bayonet and hand grenades.' I knew she was right. It was highly improbable that anybody would go to the trouble of issuing an open invitation to a party of soldiers. I bustled her and the other walking patients who had come to inspect the island into the San. doors before they started asking any more awkward questions.

The ward I was on still showed signs of the damage done to it by the bomb in the apple tree. Some hasty renovation work had been done but there was a lot less plaster on the ceilings and walls than there had been before and there was more three-ply and mesh in the window frames than glass. In the garden outside was a large hole where the apple tree had been and the flower beds would need a great deal of hard work done on them before they bloomed again.

The sister in charge of the ward was still a staff-nurse

when we went off to our country retreat. She had stayed behind to work long and terrible hours among the men from Dunkirk, and later with the casualties that were brought down from London during the Blitz. And also to earn her promotion. She was a bit self-conscious and aware of the importance of her new uniform but not too puffed up by it to scorn the cup of tea I made for her when the worst of the reorganizing was over and we could safely leave the juniors to battle on with the dirty work. The fact that she was now the ward sister did nothing to stop her glancing fearfully over her shoulder occasionally to make sure the sister wasn't creeping up to catch us at it. Drinking tea in the kitchen was as forbidden as it had always been. And just as enjoyable. The spice of the sinning added flavour to the tea leaves.

I waited until we had got through two cups each before I asked the question that had been puzzling me since I climbed down from the ambulance. Despite the familiarity of the shared tea it took courage to ask. However new a sister was she was still a sister and liable to turn nasty at a moment's notice.

'What are annexes?' I asked, then stood back an inch or two waiting for her to revert to type and tell me off for drinking tea in the kitchen and asking silly questions. She did neither. Instead she filled our cups again.

'They are wooden huts that are being put up in the field where the soldiers used to be,' she said, quite nicely. 'They are only temporary things and as soon as the war is over they will be pulled down and a proper hospital built instead.' She had no way of knowing that the annexes would be there long after the war was over, and long after they were no longer fit to be used as wards. Building new hospitals wasn't something that could be done in a hurry. We emptied the teapot and went back into the ward to shout at the juniors.

It was not till the next day that I got a proper look at the annexes. They were very functional. That night I was down on the notice board for Annexe Two.

'Where's Annexe Two?' I inquired loudly. We were in the dining-room having our evening meal before we went on nights. Nobody answered. Nobody was happy. This didn't surprise me. The first night of going on nights had never been noted for its blithe spirit. The upheaval ruined digestion, tempers and all goodwill to men and fellow-nurses. I asked again. This time with better results.

'If it's Annexe Two it must be somewhere near the end,' said someone wearily, while she sorted out a small scrap of meat from the gristle on her plate.

'Which end?' I asked, trying to make the question as conciliatory as I could. She was not conciliated.

'The end farthest away from the other end, of course,' she said. There was a short silence while she grappled with the gristle. Then, with slightly better grace, she abandoned the gristle and turned to me. 'It's the end nearest to the pub on the corner. You'll have to start out ten minutes earlier than you would if you were on the San. It's a long walk down there.' She sounded very smug. She could afford to be, she was working on the San. and had only to step outside the dining-room door to be almost on duty. 'You'll need a couple of cardigans under your cloak,' she sang out as I slouched away. 'It's bloody cold down there.' I hadn't got a couple of cardigans to put under my cloak and even if I had there was no time to go across to the home and rummage for woollies. I joined the disconsolate group who were outward bound for the annexes.

Annexe Two was Male Surgery. The sister was as new to me as I was to her. She looked at me with instant hatred. 'You're new,' she said accusingly. I admitted to the charge, adding that though I might be new to her I had been a nurse at the hospital before either she or the annexes had arrived to become blots on the landscape. I didn't exactly say any of this. Such bold statements came under the heading of 'things I would like to have said if only I'd had the courage'. What I actually said was much less forceful.

'Yes, Sister,' I mumbled apologetically. 'But I'm only new on here. I was working on the San. when the gardener found the bomb in the apple tree.' The apology did nothing to endear me to her. The fact that I had escaped unscathed from the emergency lowered me even more in her eyes. She would have appreciated me better if I had emerged from the ordeal minus a leg or two, or even a head. She had no patience with those who had nothing to show for their war effort. She had no patience with some who had.

When we had finished reading the report she took me on a round of the ward. I soon saw that her contempt for a man who had never worn a uniform was almost matched by her adulation of those who had. However little glory they may have brought to the uniform.

The patient in the first bed was swathed in bandages that enclosed his head, his arms, his chest and as much of the rest of his body as I could see from where I stood. The sister glanced fleetingly at the welter of bandages. 'Conscientious objector,' she said and looked away hastily. I stared at her and back to the man in the bed who was an object lesson in the ancient Egyptian art of wrapping mummies.

'I'm sorry, Sister,' I said, 'I'm afraid I don't quite understand.' The sister gave a snort of impatience and walked away from the bed.

'Conscientious objector,' she repeated tersely. 'Something hit him while he was doing his conscientious objecting job. Smashed his skull and broke a lot of bones.' We went on our way.

I learnt later that the young man who suffered such terrible injuries when something mechanical slipped and hit him had suffered almost as much with a conscience that refused to accept that killing for one's country was less of a crime than killing for any other reason. He bore his pain with fortitude, no doubt buoyed up by the thought that it mightn't have been any worse if it had been inflicted on him by a *Luftwaffe* pilot, a Jerry infantryman or the commander of an enemy submarine. When he was rushed to the ward with his brains not quite in the place they should have been the surgeons treated him just as if he had been a soldier and not a conscientious objector at all. They did an excellent job on restoring the brains to their original position which pleased everybody. The sister remained tight-lipped to the end.

Sitting up in the next bed, looking the picture of blooming health, was a large beefy young man. He had a red face and a mop of flaming red curls to match. The sister stood and gazed at him with affection oozing from her eyes. She tenderly patted one of his large hairy hands then stroked his curls and did up the top button of his pyjama jacket. 'And this is Andy,' she breathed. I looked at Andy and he spent a few seconds weighing me up. When he had satisfied himself that I would be putty in his hands he leered at the sister. She gave him another little pat.

'Andy is one of our dear brave fighting boys,' she murmured, her face suffused with emotion. I looked at the dear brave fighting boy and he met my eye fearlessly. 'He has been with us for quite a long time,' the sister went on fondly. There was a pause.

'What is he in with?' I asked. The sister glared at me. The insensitivity of the question had ruined the moment for her. It was an intrusion into something that was obviously something terribly personal between her and Andy. When it began to seem as if any diagnosis of the complaint that had brought Andy in was to be lost in an atmosphere of mutual adoration the sister replaced her tender look.

'We still have a few little things that need investigating, do we not, Andy?' she said. 'Too bloody right we do,' said Andy reaching into his locker for a cigarette. The sister leapt forward, grabbed a box of matches and applied a light to the Player's Weight that dangled from Andy's mouth. 'Naughty Andy,' she said, wagging a roguish finger at him. 'We're smoking out of hours again, are we not?' This time the thirteen stones of fearless manhood didn't bother to reply. He settled himself back on the pillows that the sister had plumped up for him and shut his eyes. As we moved away from the bed I glanced quickly back at him. He anticipated the glance, opened his eyes and winked at me, then closed them again. The wink admitted me into the conspiracy against the sister and against the forces that were intent on getting him back into the Forces.

'We must always remember that it is boys like Andy who are sacrificing their lives to make this a country fit for heroes,' she said, throwing a final passionate look at the sacrificial lamb in the bed. I didn't have to be reminded. From the bit I had seen of Andy he wasn't likely to be doing anything as headstrong as sacrificing his life for anybody. At least, not while he was able to conjure up symptoms sufficiently obscure to defy diagnosis. He spent most of his days thinking up fresh aches and pains to puzzle the doctors. He read articles in newspapers about men who shot off a toe or two to escape going back to the front and when somebody told him that a burst eardrum could go a long way towards getting an honourable discharge from the Army he borrowed textbooks from us in order to learn more about eardrums and ways of bursting them without causing himself too much inconvenience. He developed vague discomforts in inaccessible areas and could send the mercury in a thermometer to fever point by rubbing it briskly with a blanket while nobody was looking.

And when he wasn't busily employed with any of these things he was being incredibly helpful to us and kind beyond measure to the conscientious objector. Every morning he put himself on voluntary fatigue duties, giving out early teas, doing the breakfasts almost single-handed and rushing to get bedpans and bottles if somebody wanted one urgently enough and we were too busy to stop whatever we were doing. He was half a dozen extra pairs of hands to the nursing staff. Except when a doctor threatened to visit the ward. At the mere mention of a doctor's visit Andy got smartly back into bed and lay back on the pillows with a pained expression on his face.

The conscientious objector was even more grateful to Andy than we were. At every mealtime the reluctant hero would get out of bed and search diligently among the faceless young man's bandages for spaces to pour milky drinks through. He read out spicy bits from the Sunday papers, presumably to give the man in the bandages an urge to get out of them as fast as he could, and he told him a dirty joke whenever he could think up a fresh one – which was often. Without Andy the conscientious objector would have found life far more tedious than it was. We came to the conclusion that much of Andy's good works were done as expiation for any guilt complex he might have had.

When the sister had finished taking me round the main ward we approached the side ward. She halted for a moment, drew in her stomach muscles, threw out her bust and tapped very timidly on the door. From within came a feeble voice inviting us to enter. We entered.

The small ward had been made to look like a miniature War Office. There were official-looking documents strewn everywhere and the walls were hung with several well-pressed, much-bemedalled bits of uniform that proclaimed their owner to be a person of some importance in the field of battle – if not exactly in the battlefield.

Reclining languidly in the bed was a young man

wearing a pair of brightly coloured silk pyjamas. Beside the bed, standing stiffly to attention, hand poised in case a quick salute was called for, stood a corporal. Across the bed and carefully arranged so that not one inch of sheet or blanket should make contact with the middle region of the patient's anatomy there was a very large bed-cradle. My heart leapt. From the placing of the cradle I deduced that I was at last to have the privilege of meeting one of our brave boys who if he had not quite sacrificed his life for his country had at least donated a valuable organ for the cause. He raised a pale hand in greeting and the corporal gave the salute he had prepared himself for.

'Good evening, Sister,' said the patient wanly. The sister went scarlet. She threw herself at the bed and began to do unnecessary things to the counterpane. When she had recovered some of the composure she had lost at being addressed by so august a personage she came to attention and stood as stiffly as the corporal.

'Good evening,' she whispered. 'And how are we this evening?' The patient said nothing but gave a meaningful sigh. Taking this to be an indication that he was sinking fast I darted forward and pressed a glass of barley water to his lips. He waved it away, spilling most of it down the front of his pyjamas. The sister gave me a furious look and I mopped up the damage. The corporal again saluted and started to speak.

'Well, Miss,' he said, keeping his eyes firmly fixed on the wall opposite. 'If you'll excuse me saying so, Miss, but we're not quite ourselves today. Our – well, you know, Miss – our – well – it's been giving us a bit of pain today.' The sister uttered a cry of alarm. She steeled herself to draw down the bedclothes and I stepped forward to inspect whatever there was to inspect. There was very little. Disappointed, I stepped back again. The sister made some slight adjustment to a piece of strapping and replaced the bedding. After she had done a small genuflection in the direction of the bed we left the room.

I waited until we were well away from the side ward before I made any comment. The comment I made was not well received.

'He left it a bit late to be circumcised, didn't he, Sister?' I said. She turned on me in fury. 'Kindly remember, Nurse, that we are discussing an officer and a gentleman,' she said sharply. I accepted the rebuke and we went on our way, giving the conscientious objector another fleeting glance as we passed his bed.

When I read his case sheet later in the night I discovered that the officer who was indeed a gentleman was shortly to be married. Mercifully, during a routine inspection somebody had pointed out to him that he had a problem which if not attended to could play havoc with the mating game and cause his bride a good deal of frustration. He had done the wisest thing, though I still secretly thought that it was a bit late to start making structural alterations to his person. Especially voluntary alterations. Things like circumcision and mumps were best got over in childhood.

The junior who was waiting for me in the kitchen when I eventually got there was unlike any junior I had met before. All the juniors I had ever known were as I had been when I was a junior, timid shrinking creatures scurrying from ward to ward to be of service to their seniors and going at breakneck speed to be where they were wanted at the precise moment they were needed. To be anywhere else could get them into a lot of trouble.

There was nothing about the junior that stood at the kitchen door remotely like those juniors. She was neither timid nor shrinking. She was a large middle-aged woman, built to last, and wearing a white coat with no epaulettes or any other distinguishing badge. She smiled broadly when she saw me.

'I thought the old cow was never going,' she said, leading the way into the kitchen. 'For God's sake come and drink your tea before it gets cold.' I opened my mouth to say things about junior nurses preceding their seniors through doors and about the disrespect of calling the sister a cow of whatever age but she wasn't listening. She was too busy pouring out the forbidden tea.

'Brown,' she barked. Since the tea was more black

than brown I could only assume she was introducing herself.

While we were drinking the tea I discovered that I had a 'junior' who was senior to me in years and experience. The experience was not to be measured by the number of exams she had passed – 'Never got round to sitting for any,' she told me with a trace of regret in her voice – but by the years she had spent devotedly nursing the sick in their own homes and in small hospitals that were not training schools. I wasn't sure at first how to respond to this entirely new idea of a junior' but very soon I was giving her the respect she had earned and treating her as a nurse who though not trained knew more about nursing than I would ever know. Not perhaps the techniques of sticking needles into people or measuring out drugs but the subtle art of being able to say the right word at the right time with exactly the right amount of kindness and understanding. This was something that being State Registered wasn't always enough to qualify a nurse for. Brown was everything a nurse should be and with the war she was being given a chance to prove it.

After the tea she got up from the table and sorted out the night's work. She asked for no help from me with the sorting. She assigned the drudgery to herself and the more responsible work to me. The system worked well, though through some subtle manoeuvring on her part I often found myself sharing the drudgery with her while she helped me with the responsibility. She did it all with the sure touch of a born nurse. I only ever once saw her put out by anything and that was when she couldn't find the larder.

Because we were new to the annexes it had been necessary for the sister to take us both round and show us where we would find linen, bottles and bedpans and all the other impedimenta we would be needing.

When the first rush of work was over and the men started clamouring for their bedtime drinks Brown took the orders and went off to the kitchen to get the trolley ready. Suddenly the clattering of cups and saucers stopped and after a while I realized that operation drinks had come to a dead end. I went to the kitchen to find out what had gone wrong with the routine. Brown was standing with a mystified look on her face.

'What's wrong?' I asked her. She turned to me with some relief.

'You're never going to believe it but I've lost the larder,' she said, breaking out into a laugh. I stared round the kitchen and back at her.

'It must be in here somewhere,' I said. It wasn't. On all other wards the larder was an integral part of the kitchen but in this kitchen there was definitely no sign of a larder. There was a broom cupboard with mops and brushes that fell out the moment the door was opened. There was a cupboard under the sink which as well as housing dirty floorcloths, smelly buckets and bald scrubbing brushes was also a retreat for silverfish and cockroaches. There was a cupboard above the sink piled high with broken crockery awaiting replacement day and another cupboard full of crockery, cracked, chipped and stained but still in regular use. There was a table with a drawer in it containing a collection of cutlery that formed a breeding ground for a million different germs, but nowhere was there a larder.

'It must be somewhere on the corridor,' I said at last. We went out on the corridor. We opened doors, peered into corners, and ferreted through bathrooms taking in the usual offices on the way, but there was no larder anywhere.

We had just begun to get a bit hysterical when Andy walked out of the ward with a fag in his mouth and a glass of foaming stout in his hand. In his usual foxy way Andy had managed to persuade a junior houseman that stout was just the thing for whatever he was suffering from. Since nobody yet knew what he was suffering from he could have been right so the young houseman wrote him up for a nightly glass of stout.

'Lost something then, have you?' he said cheerfully. Feeling a bit silly, we explained about the larder. He listened sympathetically then led us out of the inner corridor door into a small vestibule between the inner and the main outer door. And there, tucked away by some maddening architect in a place where nobody would ever have thought of looking, was the larder. I was just about to thank Andy when Brown broke in. 'Why couldn't you have come sooner?' she said irately. 'You knew all the time what we were looking for, didn't you?' Andy nodded. 'Just thought I'd make you sweat for a bit,' he said and wandered back to bed.

When it was time for me as the senior to go to first midnight meal I looked despairingly at Brown. 'How do they expect us to go all the way to the main block, have a meal and get back here in half an hour?' 'We have to bike there,' she said helpfully. 'But I haven't got a bike,' I said, resigning myself to having no meal either. 'Then you'll have to borrow mine,' she said kindly.

Brown's bicycle was an elderly rusty machine with a saddle that tilted backwards the moment any weight was put on it. I was weight. I found myself sitting on the rear mudguard so often during the ride to the dining-room that the meal was down to the last scrapings when I got there and it was already time for me to set out on the return journey. The way back was made more difficult by a head wind that had sprung up. In the struggle with the elements my long black cloak slipped off my shoulders, down my legs and became enmeshed in the bicycle chain. I finished the course wearily dragging everything behind me. Brown met me at the door, clucking in a motherly way.

'There now,' she said sadly. 'I ought to have warned you. You need to tie your cloak round your waist while you're riding a bike, especially when there's any wind. Never mind, dear, we'll get Andy, he'll soon put things right for us.' She hurried off into the ward and I could hear Andy protesting at being wakened in the middle of the night and her reminding him that if he was where he should be, in foreign parts fighting for his country, he wouldn't be getting much sleep anyway. He came to the kitchen bleary-eyed and grumbling. Brown put the kettle on.

After Andy had buckled several knives and forks getting the cloak out of the chain he drank the tea Brown made for him and she secured the cloak round her waist with several large safety pins and went off for her supper. I noticed she stood on the pedals rather than risk the saddle. While she was away a most curious thing happened to me.

Before we went on duty that evening we had heard on the wireless about a convict who had escaped and was said to be armed and dangerous. None of us had dwelt too much on it at the time. It wasn't wise to dwell on such things just before going on night duty, the thought of them tended to return as the night grew longer and tiredness set in.

When I heard a door open on the corridor and saw nobody walk into the ward I immediately knew that it was the armed and dangerous convict come to do whatever was his particular weakness. I froze in my chair waiting for him to stride through the door brandishing a gun. When he didn't I was all the more frightened. A real man with a real gun I might have coped with but the terror waiting for me in the corridor was more than I could bear. I looked across at Andy. He had either already dropped off or was doing a very good imitation of a sleeping man. It seemed unfair to wake him again after he had been so good about the bicycle chain. Comforting myself with the thought that the 'thing' on the corridor might only be a gust of wind that had blown the door open, I braced myself and stepped not too boldly on to the corridor. There I froze again. It was not a gust of wind. It was a man. He was lying on the floor with his body pressed to the wall. Not an armed and dangerous criminal bent on mowing me down like a dog as the criminals on the films do, but a very old man looking more like a bundle of rags than a living human being. He looked up at me and I looked down at him.

'Good evening,' I said politely. 'Can I help you?' He appeared slightly bemused by my greeting. He drew his tattered garments around him and leaned forward to get a better look at me. I leaned back to get a more distant smell of him. After he had taken a close look at my legs he spoke.

'You're new on 'ere, ain't you?' he said, putting almost as much hatred into the accusation as the sister had earlier that night. He took a dirty piece of rag from his pocket and blew his nose. I had noticed that his nose hadn't had a good blow for a long time.

'Where's that young chap what usually lets me in?' he asked. I thought fast. There was only one young chap who would do a thing like that.

'Do you mean the one with the red hair?' I said, shrinking away from the slipstream of his breath. The old man nodded and wiped the residue from his nose down his tattered coat sleeve. 'That's 'im,' he said. 'You go and get 'im. 'E'll see me all right, Miss.' I went and got Andy. He didn't seem at all surprised when I told him there was a visitor for him outside in the corridor. He got up at once and took a brown paper bag from his locker. Then he went to the old man and gently led him down the corridor and into one of the bathrooms. He pushed the bag into his gnarled hand and shut the door.

'He'll be all right there until the morning,' said Andy. 'He only comes in when the weather's too bad to sleep rough. The chaps in the ward save the grub they can't eat for him.'

When I told Brown about the lodger in the bathroom she also wasn't as surprised as I'd expected her to be. It occurred to me that she knew all about the ward being turned into a doss-house by Andy. In the morning we shut our eyes and ears to the comings and goings down the corridor and tried not to collide with Andy and his mugs of tea and plates of bread and marge. The old man had gone by dawn but there was a lingering smell that told us he had once slept there.

When Andy at last ran out of things to confuse the doctors with they sent him back to the Army and we never saw the old man again. We missed his coming as much as we regretted Andy's going.

But soon there was more to think about and grieve over than a healthy young man with red hair or a sad old man in rags. Davies and I got news that brought the war to a terrible nearness for both of us.

Part Four

Chapter Thirteen

WHEN THE BLITZ had wreaked its vengeance on London and gone off to do terrible things to other places we, in the comparative safety of our safe area, settled down to a life of organized disorder. Sirens went and All Clears sounded, with nothing very dreadful happening in between, at least not to us, though others were still suffering the occasional horror not too far away from us. We heard bursts of gunfire as enemy planes approached and watched searchlights flare up in the night skies, then die down again until the next flare-up. Even the distant thud of falling bombs didn't scare us as much as it had before. It had all become part of living, like clothing coupons and dried egg powder. Neither of these caused us too much personal hardship. We had never enough money to buy the things the coupons entitled us to and the egg powder couldn't be tasted when it was mixed with the other tasteless delights we got in the dining-room. Being resident we escaped many of the trials that were besetting people outside. We heard about them when the visitors came.

'No eggs again today,' they grumbled furiously – or it could be biscuits, or oranges, or a more basic necessity like soap. 'Bloody grocer keeps them under the counter for his favourites. There ought to be a law against it.' There was a law against it. There were laws against almost everything, but, like the rules we were supposed to keep, they could be got round by knowing who could be bribed and what sort of bribe to offer.

The man down the road with the allotment would see the butcher right for potatoes, on condition that the butcher saw him right for a mutton chop now and then. Until the last ration book was thrown into the dustbin, or kept as a souvenir, grocers, butchers and most other purveyors of merchandise kept the choicest bits of their merchandise for the favoured few. Once rationing began it paid to become one of the favoured as quickly as possible, thereby ensuring that if there wasn't enough of something to go round, one would at least get a taste of what there was. The cooks at the hospital were nobody's favourites. Our food was at all times of the most meagre, unaugmented by any under-the-counter handouts.

But in spite of the small aggravations we were being made to endure – sugarless tea and bran scattered over everything; fire-watching when we would rather have been in bed; the occasional stick of incendiaries to keep us on our toes; and stumbling and fumbling our way in the dark with no torch batteries in the shops to replace the old ones – we were still foolish enough to think that the worst might be over for us, and there were better things in store. We went on being foolish until Davies got the letter telling her that Archibald had been taken prisoner in one of the countries his heavily censored mail had come from.

She read it many times before she allowed herself to believe a word it said. Then she sat down and read it again to make absolutely certain that what it said wasn't some terrible nightmare. When she could no longer see the words for tears I took the letter from her and read it for myself. I found it almost as impossible to believe as she had.

Though I had always known that Archibald was someone of some importance I wasn't aware of how important he was. I knew that soldiers, sailors and airmen were liable to be killed or taken prisoner at a moment's notice but that someone who was none of these things could suffer the same fate had a mystery about it which puzzled me greatly. I waited until Davies had recovered a little before I tried to get to the bottom of the mystery.

'But why?' I asked her. 'Why Archibald? He's not in the Services so why should he have been taken prisoner?' She looked at me through tear-blurred eyes.

'I think it's *because* he's not in the Services that he's been taken prisoner,' she said and looked down at the letter again.

'But what could he possibly have been doing for them to capture him?' I said, when she had stopped crying. I had no way of comforting her. The years I had spent learning how to nurse people hadn't automatically made me any better at comforting them. That was something that only came naturally to women like Baker and Brown. Either of them would have been better at coping with Davies's tears than I was.

'I don't know,' she replied. 'He never talked to me about what he did. I think it was something he wasn't allowed to talk about.' After that I asked no more questions. I saw that she had no intention of allowing her careless talk to interfere with Archibald's life, even if it was only me she was talking to and not an enemy agent.

I was to learn no more about Archibald until the day I went with Davies and stood outside Buckingham Palace while she walked in proudly to watch him being given his medal. But by that time he was a changed man, and not at all like the Archibald I remembered. He was thin and bent, and still tortured by the pain he had suffered while he was a prisoner in an enemy camp. The tributes to his bravery filled as many columns in *The Times* as the obituary notice had when his aristocratic old aunt died after Davies's devoted nursing. I watched him as he leaned on Davies's arm and saw at last all that she had seen in him that I had missed.

After the letter came Davies became quieter than she

was before. However much I tried rousing her from her apathy she sank back into it almost at once. The only time she seemed reasonably content was when she was working. She threw herself into caring for the patients with a fervour that obliterated everything else while she did it.

I watched her sad face but had only a vague idea of the things she was thinking. Though London had burned, bombs were still dropping and planes came hurtling from the skies the war had still brought me no sense of personal loss. I had pitied Bella and wept a little for her children, and felt a deep sadness when the visitors came down from London with their stories of death and destruction, but I had never had cause to mourn for anybody close to me. Then I also got a letter. It was from Baker and addressed to me, though it was intended for Davies as well. I read it as often as she had read hers before I began to weep.

'Dear both of you,' Baker had written. 'I am writing this for poor Weldon. She is beside herself with grief. Harry was killed last week. He was home on leave when it happened. A bomb fell on his mother's house while they were all sleeping. Weldon and I were on nights otherwise we would have been there as well. Think of poor Harry going through all those dreadful abroad things then coming home to be killed.' There was a postscript to the letter. 'I suppose you've heard what happened to Coventry? There's nothing left of where we used to live but thank God they were all in the shelters so at least they're alive, though a lot of their neighbours aren't.'

I tried to think of Harry going through the abroad things and coming home to be killed, but all I could think about were the days when I was his girlfriend and his mother opened tins of best red salmon for our Sunday tea, and gave us three sorts of cake laid out on a three-tiered cakestand. I thought of the little sister who had sat at the piano playing excerpts from Gilbert and Sullivan, and choruses from *Sacred Songs and Solos*. It was a long time before I could think of them as dead, and when I did there was plenty for me to weep about. At last I was able to understand a little of Davies's desolation and no longer tried telling her that she should forget her troubles and remember there were others worse off than herself. I learnt that there can be times when nobody is worse off than yourself. While the pain is fresh it takes courage to admit that others may be suffering just as much. Some never get round to admitting it.

We had indeed heard about Coventry. One visitor came to tell a patient that she was the only one left to visit her from Coventry. She told us things that haunted us for a long time after. It was easy to see that the loss of a beautiful cathedral meant less to her than the loss of so many other things she had held dear. Yet the shell of the cathedral would remain long after other shells had been removed, reminding the patient's visitor, and Baker's parents, of the way it was for them while the battle raged.

Whether because of the news about Harry and his family, or because the war was arousing feelings in me I had never felt before, I had a sudden urge to do something I had vaguely promised myself I would do someday. I told Davies what I intended doing while we were riding our bicycles along a lane one wintry afternoon. We had scrimped and scraped to buy a rackety old bicycle each. Both of them put together wouldn't have made one decent machine but we were glad of them when we were on the annexes. They got us to the dining-room on time more often. Unless some mechanical fault arose along the way.

'I'm going to London on my next day off,' I said, riding alongside her. She almost wobbled into the grass verge with shock. When she had righted herself she caught up with me again.

'What on earth are you going there for?' she asked. 'They are still dropping bombs on it and you'd be terrified if the sirens went while you were there.' I had thought of all she said and nothing had altered my mind.

'I'm going to find the house I was born in,' I shouted. She jumped off her bike and waited for me to do the same. She looked very surprised.

'But I thought you said you came from Lincolnshire,'

she said, after I had swerved to a brakeless halt beside her.

'I do come from Lincolnshire,' I said. 'But that doesn't mean I had to be born there.' She looked at me closely to see if I was joking. When she saw that I wasn't she changed the look to one of puzzlement.

'But how did you get all the way from London to Lincolnshire?' she asked, as if the distance between the two points was so enormous that miracles would have had to be done to get me there. I wasn't sure myself how I had actually made the journey, I wasn't sure of anything to do with my earliest beginnings. It was only the day before I went to be a nurse that my mother had broken the news that she wasn't my mother. Neither was my father my father. She had gone into no great detail. As in her letters she only mentioned the things I had to know and left the rest to my imagination. Not having a very vivid imagination I accepted the things she told me and had never sought to learn more. I had adjusted to an entirely different name at a moment's notice and as far as I could tell had suffered no lasting psychological traumas. Though maybe in those days there were less to suffer. Knowing about such traumas is often the surest way of becoming afflicted by them. Since I was off in the morning to be a nurse there was more for me to think about than a little thing like a complete change of identity. How I got from here to there or from there to here had never bothered me in the way it was doing now.

'I was adopted when I was a baby,' I told Davies, as bleakly as my adoptive mother had told me. Davies sighed deeply and looked at me with greater respect. For a moment her mind was diverted from Archibald, which gave the diversion at least a little therapeutic value.

'I do think it's romantic,' she said. 'When I was at school I went about pretending that I was adopted. I used to tell terrible lies about having a rich father who deserted my mother and left her to starve, so she put me in a basket and deposited me on somebody's doorstep. Were you deposited on somebody's doorstep?' I told her I strongly doubted it. Stripped of its romance my adoption was likely to have been more prosaic than a whimpering little bundle abandoned on a doorstep. Davies lost interest after that and got back on her bicycle.

'Will you come to London with me if we can get our days off together?' I shouted. She looked back at me, shaking her head.

'No,' she yelled. 'I couldn't face those moving staircase things again. And besides, you never know, you might want to be by yourself when you get there, particularly if you find the place.'

I realized she could possibly be right. It might be better to visit the place of one's birth alone. Especially in my case, when departure from it must have caused my poor young mother a certain amount of unhappiness. Having no husband to share me with couldn't have been easy for her. Not in those days when people called a spade a spade and there was a stronger word for a love-child.

On my next day off I said goodbye to Davies and set out early to catch a train to London. The day was a memorable one.

Chapter Fourteen

SETTING OUT EARLY was the first of many mistakes I was to make before I got back that night. If only I had delayed the start for an hour or two I might have spared myself at least some of the sights that were to sadden me for a long time. But since I was a true provincial at heart London for me was still a far distant land and going to it a very special and daring thing to do. It called for a lot of careful preparation as well as an early start.

From the moment I made up my mind to go I had worried about what I should wear to go in. The brightly coloured skirt, and the even more brightly coloured blouse that had clashed so well together when I wore them to go to the pictures in the town didn't seem nearly as compatible when I put them on to go to London. Nothing in my wardrobe was compatible. I chopped and changed, mixed and matched, and in the end nothing either mixed or matched. The clashing blouse and skirt were the best I could find.

I laddered the only pair of best stockings I had and

had to wash my only pair of gloves at the last minute, which meant wearing them while they were still wet. It would never have occurred to me not to wear them. Gloves were as necessary for a visit to London as a hat. I had no hat. After a lot of heavy-handed persuasion Davies volunteered to lend me hers. It was a red velour. She watched wistfully as I put it on. The thought of her best hat going all the way to London without her filled her with dread. I promised I would bring it back as good as new.

When the train stopped in the underground station we had stood in with the two airmen when we first came to the sanatorium I got off and immediately wished I was back on it again. The airman who had so blithely said that the station would make an excellent air-raid shelter had been proved right. I looked round at it and suddenly felt very sad.

Along each wall were rows of makeshift beds, some with children still asleep in them. Because it was morning and the All Clear had gone, men and women, young and old, were bustling about collecting their belongings ready to go back to the rest centres, or back home if there was still a home to go to.

Babies cried, toddlers wailed, mothers scolded and fathers swore. There were signs everywhere that the underground had become a nightly refuge for whole families. Remnants of meals lay around; paper bags spilled over, scattering small personal possessions on the platform; here and there were toys that had kept the children happy until they finally forgot the guns and bombs and had fallen asleep. It seemed to me a pity that there were children there, when they could so easily have been snug and warm in a bed in the country. Then I thought of Bella's children, and remembered that going to the country hadn't saved them. A man suddenly started to sing. He draped his bedding over a line between two packing cases and sang a song about hanging his washing on the Siegfried line, then he said something rude about Hitler and somebody laughed. Soon everybody was laughing. I was astonished that they could still laugh when there seemed so little to laugh about.

Nobody spoke to me, nobody even looked at me; and nobody seemed to mind me looking at them. They were used to being looked at by people off the trains, who didn't have to pack their things every night to go down to the station, and pack them again in the morning when the All Clear went. I had a sudden feeling that the world I was watching was the real world. More real than the world I had come from, with its few minor incidents and a bomb that had scarcely done any damage at all. I felt almost ashamed at having escaped so lightly. The people here were fleeing from real terror and escaping from a war that had already robbed them of things they would never get back. I was almost in tears when I left them behind and went on my way.

I braved the escalator and struggled up the stairs that led out to the street. People coming down collided with me and people going up jostled me. Everybody was in a hurry. I was glad when I got into the fresh air. I stood for a moment breathing it in, trying to replace the air I had been breathing down in the shelter. I thought that getting rid of that might get rid of some of the taste the sights had left in my mouth.

I had remembered to take my birth certificate with me to London. The district where I was born was difficult for anyone but a Londoner to pronounce. I had practised saying 'Marylebone' for a long time but it never seemed to sound right whichever way I said it. I had to ask a great many people before I found one who could tell me where I wanted to be. Most of them, like me, were foreigners, some from as far away as Scotland. They knew as little about London as I did.

Even after I was told where I wanted to be it took me a long time to get there. Some of the delays were of my own making, others were due to circumstances beyond my control.

Because it was the first time I had been to London I decided to go and have a look at Buckingham Palace. Having a look at it would give me something to boast about to Davies when I got back. Although she had never seen it the name was familiar to her and she would be amazed that I had dared to go there. Getting there was fraught with difficulties. First there were the roads. I had never seen so many in my life. They were everywhere. Crossing each of the many I had to cross caused me and a great many other people a lot of anxiety. It also created a certain amount of chaos. The moment I stepped off a pavement I heard words I hadn't heard before, spoken in a way that told me they were said more in anger than sorrow. Drivers blew their horns and came to a screeching halt within inches of me. Policemen abandoned their steady plod and broke into a run to drag me from under wheels. Bus drivers leaned out of their vehicles and forcibly reminded me that I was in Piccadilly Circus and not in the middle of a blooming field. I was grateful to them for telling me. I would never have known. The only thing I knew about Piccadilly Circus was that somewhere in the middle was a boy with an arrow, called Eros. There was now a thing in the middle heavily disguised with boarding and sandbags. Without Eros Piccadilly Circus was indistinguishable for me from any other Circus in London. There would have had to be clowns and a trapeze act to convince me it was a circus anyway.

The buses were as difficult to board as the roads were to cross. I got on more wrong ones than right ones and each had a conductor with a ready wit, most of it aimed at me. They had been bus conductors for a long time and could recognize a country cousin a mile away. When I was at last delivered as near to Buckingham Palace as a bus would take me the conductor helped me off with exaggerated courtesy. 'Give me love to their Majesties when yer gits there,' he said cheekily. I learnt later that the cheek was known as Cockney humour. I stuck my nose in the air and ignored him.

Buckingham Palace was a bitter disappointment to me. I stood gazing at it among a crowd of others who had come to gaze at it. What I'd expected to see I didn't know, but what I saw fell short of my expectations. I wasn't the only one to be disappointed by it.

'It don't look a bit like what I thought it would look,' said a voice behind me. 'I expected something a bit more flashy, with a few turrets and things, not all them windows with the blinds drawn.' I realized that I also had expected something a bit more flashy. It was the first royal residence I had seen and I had expected pomp and ceremony. I forgot that war could be as cruel to kings as it could to commoners.

The soldiers in the sentry-boxes were in khaki, and looked no different from any of the other soldiers who had come to stare at them. The bearskins and scarlet were put away for the duration.

I stood for a moment in front of one of the sentries looking at him intently, hoping that he would lower his eyes and look at me. He didn't and I moved off, feeling none of the thrills I had expected to feel on my first visit to Buckingham Palace.

The royal park I walked through from the Palace was just as disappointing. I had imagined acres of green grass where kings and queens from the past took time off before they went back to the Palace to order a few executions. Instead there were gun emplacements and air-raid shelters, with a few bomb craters here and there. Downing Street was the worst of all. Like so many other things in London the enchantment that distance lent faded rapidly on closer inspection. Only Westminster came up to my expectations. I stood on the bridge and agreed with all that Wordsworth had said about the majesty. My visit to London was suddenly lifted from disillusionment to exultation. The sad part was I would have no words to describe it to Davies when I got back.

The bus I at last got on, after asking at least a dozen people if it was the right bus, took an entirely different route from the one it was scheduled to take. I was made aware of this by the comments I heard the other passengers making. At every barricaded street it ground to a halt, went into reverse and chugged back to the point where things had started to get difficult. Just as it got under way again an A.R.P. warden would hold up his hand and keep us waiting while he told the driver at great length of other obstructions further along. At each diversion and each interruption groans went up from all round the bus. But the interruptions and diversions gave us a chance to do a bit of sight-seeing. Most of the 'sights' were bomb-damaged buildings and holes in the roads. They kept the passengers' minds off the delays and gave them something to boast about.

'My God, that must have been a bloody big one.'

'Not 'alf as big as the one they dropped down our way the other night.'

'You should have seen the one we had in the Blitz, fetched down a couple of pubs in one go. Lucky there wasn't anybody in them. It was after closing time.' Competition was rife. There was a lot of prestige to be gained from being the worst-bombed citizen in London. I kept quiet. I had nothing to boast about.

When the bus conductor came down the aisle and gave me a long and meaningful stare I immediately felt like a criminal. I was a criminal in his eyes. I was the sort of passenger bus inspectors are constantly on the lookout for.

'Thought you asked to get orf 'ere,' said the conductor. 'Show us yer ticket.' I showed him my ticket after emptying the contents of my handbag into my lap. The bus stood patiently while this was happening. The passengers were not so patient. They resented yet a further delay on the already long-delayed journey. The conductor examined my ticket and gave me another accusing look.

'You've only paid to 'ere,' he said. I looked round at 'ere. There was nothing about it to tell me that here was where I wanted to be. I apologized to the conductor and spent the next few minutes telling him that I'd had no intention of defrauding the bus company, and if that was how it looked to him I could assure him he was wrong. I almost went on my knees and begged him to let me off just this once. The longer I took declaring my innocence the less the conductor looked like believing me. It was the passengers who came to my assistance but not in a kindly fashion.

'For Gawd's sake, if you're going to get orf, get orf.' I got orf.

The moment I got off the sirens went. Like a drowning man who is said to see his whole life floating before his very eyes I saw vividly all that Davies had predicted about me being killed in London. I shut my eyes tightly and waited to die. When nothing immediate happened I opened them again. Everybody but me was behaving as if nothing at all had happened. Nobody looked as if they expected to be mown down. Nobody was taking the slightest notice of the sirens. I stood for a moment longer waiting to be killed, then, still very much alive, I walked on. When the All Clear came after a few minutes I felt no sense of relief. Since nothing had happened there was nothing to be relieved about. I began to understand how people who had seen so much were no longer afraid of things they didn't see.

When I stopped a policeman and asked him where exactly I would find the street I was searching for he looked at me for a moment before he spoke. There was something about the look that should have warned me.

'Well, Miss,' he said at last. 'The street you're looking for used to be just round this corner, but it isn't there any more.' And it wasn't. All there was round the corner was a roped-off barrier and an emptiness filled with rubble and ashes.

I sat on all that was left of a wall and tried to imagine what the street looked like when it was still there. Not being familiar with pre-war London streets I had nothing to guide me. I thought about my poor young mother and wondered whether she had felt sad when she wrapped me in a shawl for the last time and handed me over to somebody else. I felt a small sadness for her, and for everybody who had lived in the street when the bombs fell on it. Then I got up and left them and my mother among the rubble and the ashes and got to the station before the sirens sounded and the night bombers brought the sky to life again, and the shelterers back to their shelter.

Part Five

Chapter Fifteen

WHEN THE MATRON sent for Davies and me, to tell us that she needed our room for fresh staff who were coming in, and to ask us if we would kindly start making arrangements to become non-resident, I jumped at the idea, but not so Davies. I had been trying for a long time to get her to live out but she had always refused. She was happy where she was and would have stayed there for ever if the Matron hadn't issued her edict. But for me the chance of exchanging the all-female environment of the home for somewhere that was less like a nunnery, and might even occasionally throw its doors open to a visiting young man, was not to be lightly turned down. The only men allowed through the door of the nurses' home were doctors who had been called in to examine a case of gross malingering, or workmen who were sent for to investigate something else that wasn't functioning as it should.

Since the evening I went into the town alone and was brought back much later by an airman who possessed several of the qualities I had long been seeking it had become of vital importance that I attained some sort of liberation, if only to keep the airman's interest. Liberation meant being non-resident. I was only too happy to obey the Matron's wishes.

She had given us a short list of people in the town who were willing to accommodate nurses for the duration. It was at an address on the list that Davies and I arrived with our luggage one afternoon. The Matron had already done the preliminary introductions, without our help.

The house was large and shabby. It looked rather as if it might once have been the official residence of the lord of the manor. I paused for a moment before I rang the bell.

'Are you sure we've come to the right place?' I asked Davies, looking at the gabled windows and the wisteria that was almost uprooting the foundations. She brought out a piece of paper from her mackintosh pocket and checked the address. We had come to the right place. I tugged at the bell rope.

We could hear the jangling in some distant part of the house, then the door opened and a woman appeared. She was accompanied by three very large dogs.

The dogs threw themselves at us in a frenzy of greeting and the woman stood patiently waiting until the worst of the frenzy had died down. When I was able to get a good look at her through the barrage of dogs I again started to wonder if we had come to the right place. She didn't look at all the sort of woman to be taking in lodgers. She was aristocratically tall, with more angles than curves. She wore a shapeless knitted twin-set which in spite of its shapelessness still managed to retain an air of elegance. The elegance was enhanced by a string of pearls that had never graced a Woolworth's counter. She looked at us with an upward sweep of the eyebrows and Davies crept closer to me in self-defence.

'Yes?' she said, in a voice that perfectly matched the pearls.

'I'm sorry,' I mumbled when I realized that Davies wasn't going to mumble anything. 'I'm afraid we've come to the wrong house. We thought Mrs Darcy lived here.' I bent to pick up the luggage that the dogs were sniffing at like bloodhounds on the scent of something horrendous.

'But I am Mrs Darcy,' said the woman, losing a little of her chill. 'And you must be the nurses the dear Matron promised to send me.' At that moment yet another enormous dog hurled itself out of the door and landed with its two front feet on my shoulders. I braced myself and the woman smiled indulgently while the dog gave my face a thorough wash. When he was satisfied that I was clean – at least from ear to ear – he went off to do something urgent among the gnarled roots of the wisteria and the woman led us into the house.

The inside was as imposing as the outside, and just as shabby. There were faded velvets and worn chintzes everywhere. Though the upholstery was down to its last thread in parts the threads that remained were finer than any I had sat on before. The carpet gave the impression that it would have disintegrated entirely if it had been attacked with a sweeping brush. It hadn't been attacked with a sweeping brush for a long time.

When the woman had transformed one of the chairs into a throne by the simple act of sitting on it she scrutinized us closely through her gold-rimmed spectacles. What she saw must have satisfied her; she rose from the chair and showed us to our bedroom.

The room was as splendidly shabby as the drawing-room. It smelt strongly of lavender and furniture polish, with the essence of age to add interest.

The beds were neither low nor modern. They were great high structures that would give Davies a lot of trouble when she tried climbing into one. She had short legs. They could dangle even from an average bed. Hauling them to such heights promised to become an entertaining spectacle for me.

After we had finished inspecting the room we agreed that it could have been a lot worse, but we would have liked a little less Victoriana, and fewer pieces of solid mahogany to wake up to. We both approved of the rose-sprigged chamberpots that were modestly concealed beneath the beds. We were glad of them.

There were no ashtrays in the room and the chamber-pots would fill a need.

We sorted out our few possessions, then discovered by trial and error which door led to what on the many-doored landing, after which we went downstairs again.

There were now two women sitting in the drawing-room. The second was a smaller, paler version of the first we had met. She was finely pearled and as shapelessly twin-setted but had much less presence. As well as the two women there was an extremely old man who sat in a remote corner of the room talking to himself.

Mrs Darcy graciously begged us to be seated and waved a hand in the direction of the other woman.

'Miss Greene,' she said. 'My dear sister.' Miss Greene inclined her head but said nothing. Mrs Darcy nodded towards the old man.

'Our dear father,' she said. 'But pray pay no attention to him, he lost his mind when our dear mother died.' From then until the time we left Mrs Darcy's we paid no attention to the old man nor he to us. He spent his days chatting amicably to himself and his nights wandering round the house looking for a lavatory. On the occasions that he strayed into our room while searching we took it in turns to get up and steer him on his proper course. It happened often. His bladder, like his mind, was very weak.

When the introductions were over Davies and I sat on the sofa while Mrs Darcy and Miss Greene worked their way through balls of khaki wool. The occasional snoring of one of the dogs, the clacking of the needles and the old man's chatter were the only sounds in the room. As time passed I became extremely hungry. I had gone to first dinner, missed tea and was more than ready for my supper. I glanced across at the unidentifiable khaki mass that fell depressingly from Mrs Darcy's knitting needles and wondered how soon she would put it down and think of food.

'Balaclava helmet,' she said, catching the glance out of the corner of her eye. I blushed.

'For our dear boys across the seas,' said Miss Greene, clacking furiously. There was a long silence, broken as before by the dogs, the needles and the old man.

After the third rumble of my stomach both women put down their knitting.

'Supper, my dear?' said Mrs Darcy to Miss Greene. They got up and left the room. Davies, the old man and I stayed where we were. The dogs roused themselves and walked out of the door.

From somewhere in the house there rose a delicious smell of fried onions with faint undertones of some sort of meat. My stomach churned in anticipation. When Miss Greene appeared at the door to tell us supper was ready, and to lead the old man gently by the arm it was all I could do to refrain from breaking into a run.

The dining-room was beautiful. A ceiling-high sideboard was littered with silver and glass. There was a long table laid with a fine damask cloth and each place-setting had an array of goblets that promised wine which Davies and I – still strictly teetotal – would have to decline. Living out was to be all, and more, than I had ever hoped it would be. Or so I mistakenly thought.

We took our seats at the appointed places and Mrs Darcy bowed her head in silent prayer. If it wasn't silent it certainly couldn't be heard above the old man's ramblings.

When the prayer was over Miss Greene got up, went to the sideboard and staggered back with an enormous covered dish which she proceeded to place with some ceremony before Mrs Darcy. Mrs Darcy lifted the lid. There were no fried onions. There was no meat of any sort. There was a portion of poached haddock that I could have eaten with no help from anybody and still come back for more.

'Haddock, my dear,' said Mrs Darcy to Davies. Davies gratefully accepted the minute portion that was given to her and finished it in two enormous bites. I toyed a little with mine, trying to make it last longer. Miss Greene filled the goblets nearest to the place mats with water from a beautiful jug and we sipped it, hoping to swell the haddock to a more satisfying size.

When the empties had been piled on the sideboard Miss Greene brought over a glass bowl that looked as if it had been in the family for a long time. It was filled with a wobbly pink confection that I instantly recognized as blancmange.

'Shape?' inquired Mrs Darcy, waving a crested spoon in the air.

'Pardon?' I begged.

'Shape,' she repeated, looking into the bowl of blancmange.

'Thank you,' I said. She gave me some. I had never heard blancmange called shape before. The splendour of the name did nothing to improve the flavour of the pudding. We had it for supper every night, and in a wide variety of colours. But whether it was pink, lime green, yellow or just plain white it all tasted equally horrible.

While we were eating we could hear in the distance the sound of voices. Occasionally a dull thud or a piercing shriek penetrated the thickness of the panelled walls. When an extra loud thud was followed by a shout of laughter I looked questioningly at Mrs Darcy. Though the house was old enough for ghosts they had a reputation for stillness. There was nothing still about the noises we were hearing.

'Evacuees,' she said tersely, answering the unspoken question. 'Billeted in what were once the servants' quarters. We thought it best to live our separate lives. The arrangement suits all of us very well.' I could see that it would. The odour of fried onions wasn't at all compatible with the elegance of the meal that had just been served to us. Small it may have been, but it lacked nothing in upper-class quality.

When supper was over Mrs Darcy and Miss Greene went back to their balaclavas and Davies and I did the washing-up. This was a chore we had brought on ourselves, but the kitchen was cosier than the drawing-room and we felt more at home in it.

When we put our heads round the door to say good-night we had intended going straight to our room. Instead we followed our noses until we came to the part of the house that was once the servants' quarters. There we found the evacuees and the fried onions. There were two women and three small children sitting at a bare scrubbed table. The children were bright eyed and tidily dressed. In front of each of them was a plate with a large piece of meat liberally garnished with onions. A basin of mashed potatoes and another of sprouts were being passed around. At the end of the table was a baking tin overflowing with purple grapes and rosy apples, and a large dish of eggs. We looked at the food and the evacuees looked at us. Remembering our manners just in time, we apologized to them for inter-rupting their meal. The women said they didn't mind at all and told us to sit down and make ourselves comfort-able. Whether in answer to our eager and hungry look, or through some inborn London friendliness we were not sure, but within minutes we were sitting at the table with a plateful of steak and onions in front of us. There was as much as even I could eat. There was plenty more the women assured us, if we wanted more. It seemed they catered for any casual diner who cared to drop in.

We asked no embarrassing questions about how they had so much to offer when the meat ration was a scant half-pound per head per week. We didn't need to ask. The women were only too delighted to tell us. Their husbands both had jobs in London that made the acquisition of a pound or two of best steak a simple matter, causing nobody too much inconvenience. Steak was but one of the many choice cuts that fell from the backs of the delivery lorries when they hadn't been loaded too carefully. We were all duly grateful for the careless ways of the loaders and the blind eye of the checkers. Except Davies, and she looked slightly shocked, but she still ate.

After that it became part of the pattern of our night life to eat our *hors d'oeuvres* with Mrs Darcy and her household, wash up, then slip away for a five-star main meal with the evacuees. Mrs Darcy and Miss Greene were very pleased that we did the washing-up and promised they would mention to the Matron what dear girls we were.

When the women in the servants' quarters felt they could trust us they let us into the secret of where the abundance of fruit and eggs came from, and also the nice fresh vegetables we had in plenty.

One evening after we had left the table, full to

bursting with liver and bacon, stewed apples and plums and plenty of grapes to follow, the two women astonished us by starting to put on coats and headscarves. They wrapped the children in shawls tied in a knot at the back, and put on pixie hoods to keep their ears warm. We stood wondering what was about to happen.

'You might as well come with us,' said one of the women, looking at us with a speculative eye. 'But mind you don't go making any noise. We don't want the old girls interfering.' We gathered that the 'old girls' were Mrs Darcy and her sister. We promised that whatever we did we wouldn't make any noise.

The children, the women, Davies and I all stepped out of the back door as quietly as mice. Davies and I had on old coats that the women lent us. They were men's coats but they kept us warm.

A bright moon lit up the garden. There had been no sirens that night so the sky was peaceful.

When we reached the fence that separated the garden we were in from the one next door the two women lifted up their skirts and climbed nimbly over. I looked at Davies and saw that she was wishing she hadn't come. It was too late for wishing. We were there.

The women threaded their way between neat rows of this and that then stopped at a tree. We could see them shaking the branches and heard the soft thud of falling fruit. Soon they were back at the fence with apples that they dropped into the children's outstretched hands. The cabbages they brought back from their next forage were crisp and fresh, and glistening with the evening dew.

'A few eggs now, and that'll be all for tonight,' whispered one of the women, unloading a pinny full of Brussels sprouts.

'We've got enough grapes to see us through to the end of the week.' Off they went again, but this time in the direction of the henhouse. For a moment we could hear the muffled sounds of protest as the hens were moved to give up the fruits of their labour. Then all was quiet again and soon everybody was standing on the right side of the fence. Davies waited until we were safely inside the house before she registered her protest.

'But surely it must be stealing,' she anxiously, while the fresh garden produce and the free-range eggs were being stacked away in the larder. The women turned in surprise.

''Course it ain't stealing,' said one of them, with a touch of contempt for Davies's scruples. 'He lives all by himself and he don't need all that lot. And he don't give none of it away neither, so we just goes in and helps ourselves.' She giggled and nudged the other woman. 'Bloody good job he's deaf and goes to bed early, ain't it, mate?' All of us, except Davies, agreed that it was. She still had some doubt about the ethics of relieving a man of his property, however reluctant he might be to part with it voluntarily.

The man next door turned out to be not everybody's favourite character. He had a reputation for meanness and had never been known to stretch out his hand to help anybody. Mrs Darcy and Miss Greene resented it strongly that by some means he had escaped having evacuees billeted on him though his house was large and his garden productive. If they knew anything about the marauding in the garden it was never spoken of, nor did they comment on the few parsnips they found on the kitchen table, or the egg or two that appeared overnight in the china hen on the dresser. Davies and I felt it was only right for them to benefit occasionally from our misdeeds. Especially since we were guests under their roof. It took Davies a little while to shake off her scruples but once she had she ate the stolen goods with as much enjoyment as if somebody had queued for hours outside a shop.

I had discovered to my sorrow that courting while I was residing in Mrs Darcy's house was no easier than it was while I was a resident in the nurses' home. There were possibly even more drawbacks to it. Though coming in late had been an unforgivable crime if we were caught, coming in late without being caught had quickly been brought to a pitch of perfection, especially when the soldiers arrived on the scene. But at Mrs Darcy's house there was no way in but the front door, and only one time to come in, which was at the stroke of ten or earlier. The back door was firmly bolted and barred at ten prompt and one or other of the two ladies took up their position at the front door to bolt it as well, once we had stumbled over the threshold. This put a stop to any dreams I might have had of prolonged goodnights on the doorstep or surreptitious creepings up the back stairs. It was very frustrating after all the hopes I had pinned on living out.

But in spite of the obstacles the courtship survived and gathered strength, and finally came to the notice of Mrs Darcy. She spent the whole of a poached haddock session questioning me about my young man's family, his background, his ambitions and any likelihood there was of his ambitions being realized. I made up most of the answers to satisfy her requirements and at last the day came when he was invited to take tea in the drawing-room.

The visit was a great success. Remembering the days when the followers of the lower orders were kept at a respectable distance until the ring was placed on the finger Mrs Darcy sat my airman and me as far apart as the seating arrangement in the drawing-room allowed, taking into consideration the old man's running commentary on something that was currently happening in the Holy Roman Empire.

When the visitor had taken his leave and rushed off to be back at camp before he was put on fatigue duties for being late Mrs Darcy turned to me.

'He seems a perfectly respectable young man, my

dear,' she said kindly. 'That will be sixpence.' I stared at her. The first part I understood but the second I didn't understand at all.

'I'm sorry, Mrs Darcy,' I said. 'I'm afraid I don't quite understand.' She seemed surprised at my obtuseness.

'But surely I made myself clear, child. I said that will be sixpence.'

'What will be sixpence, Mrs Darcy?' I asked, genuinely not knowing.

'The tea will be sixpence, of course,' she said. 'There was the buttered scone, a portion of home-made jam and a cup of tea. Actually, there were two cups of tea but we will disregard the second.' I thanked her for disregarding the second cup of tea, begged her to keep an account of my debts in a little book, and promised to settle up with her on payday.

After that, whenever the young man drank so much as a cup of tea in the drawing-room, the cost was carefully debited to my account and the total added to my living-out bill at the end of the month. I had to meet the extra financial burden myself; the hospital allowed no such things as expense accounts.

I never invited my airman for supper. I trembled to think what Mrs Darcy would have charged for his portion of shape.

Chapter Sixteen

THE BLITZ WAS over, vanquished valiantly by 'the few', but the war went on, becoming less endurable as it went on. The spirit that had made Dunkirk a victory rather than a defeat, and had kept the jokes about Hitler alive during the Battle of Britain, was at last giving way to feelings of despair. Nothing was getting any better and it had started to look as if nothing ever would. Nobody knew how it was all going to end. The optimists still declared we would win the war, but the not so optimistic had their doubts.

The visitors came down from London and sat grumbling to each other instead of chatting happily to the patient they had come to see. He didn't have to queue for his supper like they did. With fewer bombs to boast about there was more time for dwelling on other things. Heroes got no priority in the line-up for potatoes.

They grumbled about the bacon ration, the tea ration and the one egg they got a week, which was likely to have turned bad before they got it. Or so they told us. They didn't like the greyish bread they were having to buy since the enemy stepped up the attack on ships bringing in the harvest. There was no longer any virtue in making do and mending. They had done it for so long that mends were being mended and patches patched.

The poor grudged the rich the meals they could afford to eat in restaurants and the rich bemoaned the fact that by law they could only spend five shillings on the meal they ate. Some went as far as to pop out one door after a meal and pop in another for an extra five shillings' worth. There were still plenty of ways round if only you knew the proper route.

When the British Restaurant opened in the town it was a godsend to hungry nurses. Instead of having to eat their dinner in the dining-room on their days off they could go to the British Restaurant and get a slap-up three-course meal for ninepence. A great deal to eat for as little outlay as possible had been the dream of nurses for a long time. The British Restaurant was the dream fulfilled.

The news that made news was almost always bad news. The fall of Singapore had us searching a map of the world to find where it had been before it fell. Only those who came top in geography at school could find it without travelling with their finger across two continents. Tobruk fell and, except for the thousands who fell with it and their loved ones, was but another name in the newspapers.

But there were names that were familiar to every-body – even to us. Mr Churchill, Vera Lynn and Alvar Liddell were recognized on the wireless almost the moment they opened their mouths. If Vera had become the sweetheart of the Forces, then Alvar Liddell, Stewart Hibberd and Bruce Belfrage had become the voices of the people. Whether they would have stood up to the blinding light of television was something they didn't have to worry about. They could have been a bunch of hunchbacks straight out of Notre Dame so long as their bland and silky voices never faltered or trembled. Grandmas and maiden aunts vied with each other to be the first to identify the voice that said: 'This is the news and this is—', before the voice revealed who it was who was reading the news. If a stranger had sat before the microphone he would have been unmasked by millions at the first utterance.

'Lily Marlene' stood as high as 'The White Cliffs of Dover' in the top ten, and 'Music While You Work' kept the workers working and the highbrows shuddering.

Pearl Harbour had finally brought the Americans into the war and the Americans were bringing a different sort of war to the towns and villages by giving the local girls a taste of the honey they were missing while their regular boyfriends were away. The regular boyfriends said a lot of nasty things about the Americans. We didn't. We had a lot to thank them for.

When Johnny was brought into the children's ward

with a disease that could never be cured but might be helped by things that were in short supply we put out an emergency call for bananas. Bananas were the yellow, banana-shaped things that none of our children had ever seen. They had stopped appearing in the shops when their space was needed for more valuable things. But for Johnny a banana in his diet could add a year or two to his life.

It was the Americans in a nearby camp that answered the emergency call. Magically they conjured up bananas and brought them for Johnny. When they saw our children they thought of their children back home and came to see ours again. They came with pockets bulging and paper bags bursting. They brought candy for the children and things they called 'nylons' for us. The nylons were the key that opened many doors for the Americans. For a long time we believed that for the premium of a single pair of nylons our legs would be covered for life. Nylon was indestructible, they told us; there would be no more laddered stockings, and no more toes peeping through holes. None of us stopped to think that such a utopian stocking would mean the ruination of all the hosiery manufacturers. We were soon to realize that a pair of sturdy black woollen ones would outlast several pairs of nylons, which needed to be repaired by experts or thrown away after the first few wearings. Nylons were just one of the many things that didn't quite live up to the claims that were made for them.

As well as all the other little luxuries the Americans brought, they came loaded with chewing gum. This was as exciting to the children as the American accent. The novelty caught on and stuck as fast as the gum. We found wads of chewed-up putty adhering to bed-rails, glued to lockers, and clinging to the soles of our shoes. We peeled it off pyjamas, pulled it away from pillow-cases, combed it out of curls, and fumbled for it up noses and as far down as eardrums. Though we wouldn't have dreamed of associating ourselves with the slogan 'Yanks go home' we would willingly have appended our names to a petition that called for the repatriation of chewing gum. Our poorly sick cherubs sat chewing like small ruminants. As they chewed, a glazed look of contentment spread across their faces.

We might have been less tolerant with the new craze that the ward maids were scraping off the floors if there hadn't been some compensation for it. It kept the children occupied while we told them things we didn't like telling them. A stick of gum worked wonders for a child who had recently become an orphan. It temporarily took his mind off wondering why his mummy and daddy hadn't been to see him that day. The Americans were as valuable as the gum they brought. They were marvellous at filling in the gaps on visiting days. They made splendid fathers if it was a father that was missing, and could even double up as a mother if one was needed badly enough. They were as comforting as a comfort rag and as soothing as a dummy. Their role as foster-parents was sometimes taken beyond the ward doors.

When the young lieutenant came laden with goodies and saw Patsy for the first time he was captivated by her. She had sparkling blue eyes and a mischievous laugh. She had been making him laugh for quite a few minutes when she asked politely whether he would mind if she ran her hands over his face to find out what he looked like. We had forgotten to tell him she was blind. The shock of discovering it for himself was almost more than his tough American guy image could take. When he had completely recovered from the shock he got permission to send Patsy out to his child-less wife in New Mexico, the understanding being that she would stay there forever if the arrangement was satisfactory to all parties. The arrangement was most satisfactory. Patsy became one of the many children who were finding fresh roots in America.

Some of the nurses were also making preparations for becoming American citizens. They came in at night, rosy with happiness and proudly flaunting their new rings, and already wondering what to wear when they met their in-laws for the first time. The thought of them being American in-laws appeared not to daunt them at all.

Others were finding favour with the Polish airmen who had set up in opposition to the Americans and the

British at the pub on the corner. The Polish engagement rings worried me more than the American ones, though I had no idea why they should. I tried to put the worry into words one day.

'Aren't you worried?' I asked a nurse who was frantically reading up Warsaw so that she wouldn't show her ignorance when she went there.

'No, why should I be?' she asked. I said I didn't know, but wasn't it a bit risky marrying a man who wouldn't understand what you meant when you threatened to go home to your mother? The nurse laughed and assured me that he'd understand all right, she had ways of making him understand. I still wasn't convinced. But I was wrong. When the war was over there were plenty of statistics to prove that the couples who screamed at each other in the same language were as much at risk as those who hurled their abuse in different tongues.

The war that had ruined so many people's lives had passed lightly over the Darcy roof. Except for Davies, myself and the evacuees, life had gone on for the two women and their father with not too many disruptions. The greatest upheaval for them took place one night when London had at last grown quieter and the sirens were enjoying a well-earned rest. There was no scream of bombs or blinding light of incendiaries to imprint the occasion on our memories.

Davies and I were biking back to our lodgings and

looking forward to putting our feet up somewhere when we turned the corner and saw Mrs Darcy, her sister and their poor old father huddled together out on the road. We fell off our bikes and rushed across to the sad-looking trio. The women were weeping and clinging to each other while the old man did his best to comfort them with some lines from a Greek classic.

After we had managed to make sense out of the women's terrified incoherence we gathered that a vast multitude of friends and relations of the evacuees had descended on the house like a plague of locusts, bent on celebrating every anniversary that had gone neglected while the war was bringing the world down round their ears. From the noise we could hear coming through the blackout the party was going with a swing. Poor trembling Miss Greene told us that the house was packed with aunts and uncles, nieces and nephews, brothers and sisters, and a host of friends and neighbours culled from far-flung Hackney and all points east. They had come with bottles of this and crates of that and a mouth organ or two to liven things up when they looked like flagging. The strains of 'Down at the Old Bull and Bush' could clearly be heard.

Davies and I quickly got the message that Mrs Darcy and her sister were relying on us to evacuate the evacuees. The thought of doing anything so frightening made us tremble as much as they were trembling. When we saw there was no other way we propped up our bicycles against a laurel bush and crept up the garden path.

The first timid pull I gave to the bell rope brought no results. I pulled again, a decibel louder, hoping that there would still be no results. To my intense horror a window was flung open, a bald head appeared, and a voice asked us who we were and what we wanted. The question contained some vividly descriptive expletives. I left it to Davies to supply the required information. Timidly she informed the head that we lived there and we would be grateful if they would open the door and let us in and themselves out. This so incensed the bald head that it withdrew itself from the window with a few further descriptive adjectives. Davies and I went back to the group on the pavement and admitted defeat. The party went on with renewed vigour.

Both the women were beginning to lose some of their stiff-upper-lip upper-class control, while the old man was showing unmistakeable signs that the night air was taking its toll of his bladder. Something clearly had to be done before the self-control and the bladder were beyond redemption.

'I think we ought to go for the police,' said Davies at last. Miss Greene gave an anguished yelp. The road was in a select part of the town. Going for the police was something that only the lower classes did. The neighbours would have taken extreme umbrage had they seen a posse of police riding up on their bicycles. 'Not the police,' she gasped. 'I couldn't bear the disgrace.' Davies and I rejected the idea of the police and tried to think of a better one.

'I know,' I said suddenly, jabbing Davies in the stomach. 'What about Brown?'

'Well, what about her?' asked Davies when she had recovered from the jab.

'She's the one,' I said. 'She could get anyone out of anywhere. She's marvellous at getting people to do things they don't want to do.' Davies thought about Brown for a moment, then nodded her head. After a short debate which I lost I jumped back on my bike and went to get Brown.

She was already in bed with a good book. Despite her eagerness to get back into the swing of nursing after being away from it so many years she was only too glad to get her feet up at the end of a long day. They needed all the rest they could get between padding on duty in the morning and limping off again at night. When she saw me appear at the door she put down the book.

I told her as briefly as I could about the extraordinary things that were happening at our lodgings and she listened intently. When I had finished she dragged herself out of bed and got dressed at once. Then she went with me to get her bike out of the shed. Brown dearly loved a fight. She would take on anybody, whether it was a porter who failed to give her the respect she demanded or a patient who insisted on doing things for himself that Brown thought she should be doing for him. Though she hadn't had much practice at evicting evacuees she was willing to have a go.

When we got up the garden path she wasted no time on the bell rope. She hammered on the door loudly enough to make herself heard above the frenzied knees-up we could hear coming from the drawing-room. When the same bald head that had greeted me appeared at the window she didn't give it a chance to ask who she was and what she wanted. She got her say in first.

'Here, you,' she shouted at the top of her voice. 'Come down here at once and open this bloody door!' The owner of the head was so taken aback at being spoken to in language he could understand that he withdrew his head without a word and within seconds the door was opened and we were all inside. Brown strode through the hall with Davies, me and the Darcys trailing after her. The Lambeth walk that had been going so well fizzled out with the faintest of 'Oys' and the dancers stood looking uncomfortably from one to the other.

'Out,' cried Brown, flicking a thumb in the direction of the door. 'Get out this minute or I'll chuck you out.' By this time she had her coat off and her sleeves rolled up. The important-looking man who was dispensing drinks from the piano lid picked up a bottle and a corkscrew and looked at Brown with deepest respect. Had he been wearing a cap he would most certainly have raised it to her. Very carefully, to keep the froth intact, he poured out a glass of stout and handed it to her. She accepted it without thanks and emptied it in one long draught. His respect for her grew visibly.

''Old on a minute, Miss,' he said, pleadingly. 'We couldn't go now, even if we wanted. There's no trains back at this hour of the night. And besides, the kids is tired, they ain't had much sleep lately. You wouldn't be so 'ard as to chuck us out, would you, Miss?' Brown leaned over him and helped herself to another bottle of stout. Carefully she filled her glass.

'I most certainly would,' she said firmly. 'You lot thought nothing of chucking out these poor old things, did you?' The man looked at Mrs Darcy and back at Brown.

'Begging your pardon, Miss,' he said. 'It wasn't so much us as chucked them out as them not wanting to join in the party. We did ask them but they was a bit above it, like, see?' Brown saw. She drained her glass.

'All right,' she said, wiping the froth off her mouth. 'You may all stay here tonight but you must sleep where you can and let these poor old things get to bed. You ought to be ashamed of yourselves treating them like this at their age.'

I looked at Mrs Darcy, trying to see her through Brown's eyes. Until then I had never thought of her as a poor old thing, but suddenly I knew that she was. Her world had been turned upside down by the war almost as much as the evacuees' had, and unlike theirs hers would never be the same again. Theirs had a chance to be improved upon. A revolution was already starting that would make the man pouring out the drinks in his shirtsleeves as important as Mrs Darcy's learned father had ever been. Shirtsleeves were rapidly becoming invested with as much power as the whitest of white collars. Brown went on laying down her law.

'Tomorrow one of you must go down to the Advice Bureau and see if they can do anything about the children, though why you didn't have them evacuated from the start beats me.'

Davies and I helped Brown to arrange and organize until there was a place for everybody and everything back in its place then she got on her bike and pedalled furiously back to bed. I felt proud of myself for thinking of going for her. She was just what was needed in an emergency. Especially the sort of emergency that called for a sympathetic understanding of other people's needs. It was one of the best things that had happened to hospitals when they amended their rules and enrolled women like Brown into their service.

When the air-raid wardens found themselves at a loose end, with no air raids to keep them busy and no bombs to worry them, they started flashing their torches in all the secret places where courting was done before it became permissible to do it anywhere. On the third occasion that they flashed a beam in the church porch and discovered my airman and me having a little rest after a long walk back from the town we began making plans to get married. Like many other things in wartime it was easier to plan than to finalize. There were snags from beginning to end. And beyond.

Part Six

Chapter Seventeen

GETTING MARRIED IN wartime was not always easy. There were too many different parts to be assembled before a successful whole could be achieved. It often happened that one of the parts was missing at the last minute. It could be the bridegroom.

Being usually at the bidding of his king and country made it a strong possibility that he would be sweltering to death in some arid desert when he should have been shivering with cold and fright in the pouring rain outside a register office or sheltering beneath a church porch. There was seldom anything that could be done about this except scrap the plans and the forty-eight-hour honeymoon and hope for better luck next time.

It was occasionally the banns that went wrong somewhere. Either they had not been called at all, owing to a mix-up in the assembly line, or they had been called in the wrong place or at not enough places. This could sometimes be remedied by a quick dash to buy a special licence if the money in the kitty was enough to cover the cost of a special licence and all the conditions were favourable to its legality.

But even if the groom and the banns had behaved faultlessly there was still the chance that the church could have slid down a bomb crater in the middle of the night, or the best man might have sent a telegram saying he wouldn't be there and neither would the chief bridesmaid as they had decided to get married to each other while there was still time. Blessed the bride that got it all together without a hitch. Or managed to get hitched without getting it all properly together.

Getting married in wartime had its own special problems for a nurse. Her main stumbling block was often the Matron. Being mostly unmarried themselves the most understanding of Matrons found it hard to understand why a nurse should be so eager to exchange the security of being superannuated at sixty for the shifting sands of marriage. They spent long and often fruitless hours pointing out the folly of it all.

The Matron of our hospital was the kindest and most understanding of women, but she was no different from the others – of whom there were many – when it came to a request for permission to get married.

After a great deal of soul-searching and a lot of friendly advice from Davies I faltered to the office to ask if I could get married. The Matron wasn't at all sure. I had caught her at a bad time. She was still reeling from the shock of discovering that her second-in-command had crept out one morning unbeknown to any but her closest friends, and had returned to the hospital openly married to an officer from the R.A.F. camp. Since then one or two of the sisters, including the more senior ones, had been going about with a far-away look in their eyes. It had obviously only taken one to set them all off.

We had long suspected that the second-in-command was up to something. Rumour had it that the officer from the R.A.F. camp could be collided with on the drive some nights, looking guilty but fulfilled and only too willing to lend a hand with getting a nurse in late by one of the routes he used to get himself out late. The confirmation of the rumour had put the Matron in a very bad mood: no mood at all for offering me her felic-itations.

When I first went to be a nurse I had spent hours on the mat in the office being told off for things I'd done that I shouldn't have done, and things I'd forgotten to do that it was my duty to remember. I now found myself in exactly the same position. I was kept on the mat while the Matron told me off for even thinking of doing a thing that would cause her so much inconven-ience. She reminded me that there was still a war on and nurses were in greater demand and shorter supply than they'd ever been. She reluctantly admitted that it had become permissible for nurses to marry but hastened to impress upon me that the permissibility did nothing to lighten the burden of staffing a hospital. Married nurses had a habit of messing up the holiday lists and leaving gaps on the wards while they rushed away to have babies.

I was just about to promise her most sincerely that I would do nothing so outrageous when I remembered in time that messing up the holiday lists and having babies were failings I was as likely to be afflicted with as any other nurse. I kept quiet and the Matron said more.

I had begun to wonder whether getting married was worth all the trouble I was going to when the Matron suddenly capitulated and started discussing dates. After much this-ing and that-ing she finally granted me one week's leave. The week was my due, but she granted it as a favour.

The week she granted me didn't quite coincide with the few days my airman's C.O. had as reluctantly granted him, but with an overlapping weekend we could consider ourselves lucky. At least we weren't having to get married by proxy.

Davies was delighted when I told her the Matron had said I could get married. All she asked was that she could be my bridesmaid. The simple request threw me into a panic. Though we had planned on a church wedding the allotted cash hadn't allowed for extras like a bridesmaid. Having to clothe Davies as well as myself turned a latent headache into a threatened nervous breakdown. But she was very understanding when I shared the financial problem with her. We went through our wardrobes one evening and with a little from hers and a little from mine we were at last able to rustle up an outfit that wouldn't, we hoped, look too awful when she was bringing up the rear down the aisle.

I tried not to bore her too much with the details of the forthcoming event. The thought of Archibald not there to see her being a bridesmaid for the first time caused her a lot of unhappiness. But she didn't allow her unhappiness to cloud my happiness.

Mrs Darcy wasn't delighted at all. She echoed all that the Matron had said, adding a lot of extras of her own. She made it clear from the start that there would be no place for me to lay my head in her house when I needed a bridal bed to lay it on. Having me rushing up to the attic room when my airman was there, and rushing down again to share Davies's room when he wasn't, gave a touch of the illicit of which Mrs Darcy assured me her dear father would have strongly disapproved had he been of sound mind and able to appreciate anything that was going on. He had, she said, been a man of the highest principles.

Short of Davies making a threesome in the attic, or my future intended setting up a mini-harem in the room below, there seemed no way out of the dilemma but for me to find lodgings elsewhere. I promised I would see to it at once.

I studied the ads in the paper-shop window and kept

an ear to the ground until I heard about a lady who had a room to let, with a double bed, full use of bathroom and a cup of tea in bed in the morning whenever she felt like giving me one. And all for two and sixpence a week, meals extra. The cup of tea would be thrown in, she said. I gave her rent in advance and got on with the more pressing arrangements.

'Come to my wedding,' I wrote to Baker and Weldon, adding that if Weldon had still no heart for it I would quite understand. They both accepted the invitation and I included their names on the guest list. The list was very short. We were keeping it short, our financial position excluding any unpatriotic ostentation. I went and asked the lady who had got my rent in advance if she would mind Baker and Weldon using the room for an overnight stop. She said she didn't mind at all, they'd be ever so welcome bless their hearts. I thanked her from the bottom of mine.

The wedding ring and the one-tiered cake were as hard to come by as the Matron's permission to get married.

'No wedding rings,' said the only jeweller in the town. 'Can't get gold for love nor money. There's a war on, you know.'

'No fruit cake,' said the baker near to the hospital. 'Couldn't get a sultana if you was to offer me a fortune. There's a war on, you know.' With neither love for the jeweller nor a fortune for the baker I went one way looking for something to put in a cake and my airman went the other in search of a ring.

The ring was discovered at the final hour lurking in a dark corner of a shop where it had lain forgotten for a long time. With a bit of breathing on and a quick rub with a duster it was barely distinguishable from twenty-two carat.

I wasn't so lucky with the dried fruit. After tapping all the black markets that Mrs Darcy's evacuees knew I abandoned the idea and begged the baker to do his best without the benefit of sultanas and raisins.

Davies went with me to buy the bridal outfit. The day we went I was at a more than usually low ebb moneywise. There had been several hidden extras I hadn't reckoned for – things like a pair of stockings and a few cigarettes to pass round at the reception. We pooled our clothing coupons and went looking for a little number that would look lavish enough for a wedding and still leave a shilling or two over for the hat and shoes. The hat had a wispy bit of netting that partially obscured the view from my right eye. Most brides of the day had hats with a netting that partially obscured the view from at least one eye. The netting occasionally extended over both eyes which could cause trouble when there were steps to climb.

Davies insisted that she should buy the bouquet as a wedding present, thus killing two birds with one stone as it were. I gratefully accepted the offer. The resources had run out and a bouquet was rapidly becoming a wearisome financial burden. She went to a flower shop and ordered an enormous spray of trailing maidenhair fern with as many red roses and blue scabious entwined among it as she could afford. The maidenhair fern came down far enough to disguise my knees, which the dress barely reached. It was this shortness that had brought down the price enough for me to afford it.

The wedding went off very well. The only jarring note was the vicar. He had an obsession about the dry rot that was attacking his organ which drove him to rattle his begging box beneath our noses almost before the ceremony was over. He got no help with his organ from us. He also stood in the way while the photographs were being taken, insisting that not one jot or tittle of confetti should fall on his clean-swept paths. By this time a force eight gale was blowing my dress up in swirls above my waist. Without the vicar's presence this uncalled-for immodesty would have encouraged more vulgarity than it already did. My airman's best man had a keen sense of humour.

The reception was held in the pub on the corner. There was a bit of gate-crashing but nothing that we couldn't handle. Brown was there to maintain discipline. She also had gate-crashed but became such an asset that we forgave her and allowed her to stay. She was in uniform, which lent a professional touch.

The cake was delivered to a side door just when I had

begun to give up hope that it was going to be delivered at all. The man who delivered it was the man I had asked to do his best. He had.

'It's dates,' he said.

'What's dates?' I asked.

'The cake's dates,' he replied. He spoke in the tones of a man who has achieved the miracle of turning wine into water. I placed my bouquet on the floor and took the cake from him. He threw a swift glance down at my unferned knees.

'It had to be dates,' he said. 'There wasn't no dried fruit and you did ask me to do my best.' I thanked him kindly for doing his best. Nobody could have done more.

'There wasn't no icing sugar, either,' said the man. He carefully removed a paper doyly from the top of the cake. Without it the cake was brown and lumpy. He quickly replaced the doyly.

'I'd get it eaten as fast as you can,' he said anxiously. 'Egg powder ain't like the real thing and dates 'as a tendency to go off sooner than currants.' They had already gone off. The guests sat picking them out and laying the mouldy fragments round the edges of their plates, along with all the other fragments they hadn't thought much of from the cold buffet. Mrs Darcy and Miss Greene waved aside the slabs of cake I offered them and suppressed a shudder. They were used to better things.

Seeing Weldon looking pale and sad and not a bit like the Weldon I remembered made me almost wish she hadn't come at all. I thought of Harry and his family and for a moment mourned for the days when there wasn't a war to spoil things for everybody. At least not a war that had landed on our own doorstep.

Baker had got through after her own fashion; though, with the death of her brother, and Coventry, and her fears for Dr Collins who was in every fighter plane she heard had been shot down, there were shadows in her face that hadn't been there before. Nevertheless there was still plenty of spirit left in her. She glanced round at the reception with a profound look of disgust.

'My God,' she exclaimed, removing a portion of date from her mouth. 'I've tasted some rubbish in my time but this beats all.' She held up a lump of date that looked as if it had been attacked by a swarm of fruit-fly. 'As far as I can see you'll be bloody lucky if you get away with it without somebody going down with something awful.' After that I made sure my new young husband didn't eat any of the cake before I had gone over it carefully for mildew.

Weldon helped herself to a ladleful of the scummy-looking fluid in a pudding basin. She choked and went purple. 'Whatever is it?' she asked, the tears pouring down her cheeks. Davies gave her a heavy pat between the shoulders and she slowly got her breath back.

'It's punch,' I said. 'Like the stuff the Matron used to make for the hospital balls while we were doing our training.' Davies and I had gone to great pains to get the ingredients together. We had poured in a drop of this and a little of that, all strictly non-alcoholic, and at the very last minute the evacuees had given us a bottle of something they said was 'spirits'. If it was it did nothing to lift the spirits of the punch. However teetotal the guests might have been they could have polished off the lot without offending their principles. But after one sip none of them seemed to show much inclination for it. Just as none of us had shown any inclination for the punch at the hospital balls.

'It tastes worse even than the cake,' said Baker, pouring her remainders back into the basin.

I was starting to feel a little hurt at their reception of my reception, until I remembered that for all the years we'd worked together we had never been unstinting in our criticism of each other, and instead of feeling hurt I was suddenly glad that I had friends who liked me enough to be rude to me. If the ones we love are the ones we hurt then the ones we can be most rude to are surely our best friends.

My father and mother were not at the wedding. I had sent them a hand-printed invitation card, but I had known when I sent it that they wouldn't come. My father never ventured further than the local cattle market and it wouldn't have occurred to my mother to

leave him to fend for himself while she went galli-
vanting all the way to London. He wouldn't have
fended anyway – he would sooner have starved.
Cooking, like cleaning, was a woman's work and he
had never lifted a finger to do either in his life. Nor had
he been expected to. The day of men wearing pinnies
had still to come, along with women's lib.

My father-in-law had come a long way to see his only
son get married. He had travelled through the night and
was already looking tired. I sat by him while we talked,
avoiding the cake and punch, and growing fonder of
each other as we talked. He seemed to like having me
for a daughter-in-law. The liking was mutual.

'What are you doing about a honeymoon?' Baker
asked me, when I was having a break from mingling
with the guests. I thought of the day that Baker got
married and how embarrassed she was when Weldon
asked her the same question. She had blushed furiously and almost choked over the question. The war
had stopped a lot of blushing over honeymoons, and
over many other things. Blushing was definitely on its
way out. I blushed furiously and busied myself with
the bouquet for a moment. For various reasons it took
me a long time to bring myself to give them my honeymoon address. Weldon sat waiting for it with an
expression on her face that told me she was thinking
of the week she had spent in Llandudno with Harry
while I was in the sick bay having measles. I shook off

the memory of the measles and answered Baker's question.

'Well, actually, we're not going anywhere special,' I said, trying to sound as casual as possible. 'We tried everywhere, but we couldn't get in anywhere, so we're going to my mother's for the weekend.' The last bit came out in a rush. There was a sudden silence. Davies got up in a hurry and went off to try and get rid of a bit more of the cake and a drop more of the punch, while Baker and Weldon put down their plates and stared at me.

'But will he like it there?' asked Weldon at last, looking at my new husband, scrubbed and polished in his Air Force uniform. 'You know what I mean. Your mother and the lavatory and all that.' Weldon had biked home often with me while we were doing our training. She had learnt a lot about my mother. She knew also that our lavatory was round the back with nettles growing through the seat, and that we brought a tub in on Saturday nights and bathed ourselves in the kitchen. She looked again at my husband.

I assured her that on the few occasions I had taken him home he had accepted both my mother and the other rural aspects of our house without too much complaint, though I had noticed that when he went round the back he spent a few minutes arranging the lavatory door so that the train drivers didn't get an uninterrupted view of the proceedings as they did when it was propped up against the water butt which was its natural habitat.

'But you can't possibly have a honeymoon there,' said Baker. 'I thought your mother didn't believe in you-know-what. She's hardly likely to approve of a honeymoon going on under her very roof.' I blushed again. I knew that Baker was referring to things I had told her about my mother not believing in fish or sex. She had strict ideas about both. I had never seen so much as a shrimp enter our house. I wasn't too happy about taking sex into it. I got up and went over to my father-in-law who was starting to get restless.

'I'd better be getting along,' he said, looking wistfully at the son he hadn't seen for a long time, and wouldn't be seeing for a long time.

'Where are you getting along to?' I asked stupidly.

'I'm going home,' he said. It was only at that moment that I remembered I had done nothing about arranging an overnight stop for him as well as Baker and Weldon. I suddenly felt very sad.

'But you can't go home,' I said. 'You only came this morning and there won't be any trains back there tonight.' 'Back there' was a complicated journey that started in one of the great London stations and ended at a point far north. Even in peacetime the journey had taken many hours, but war had made the place almost inaccessible. The thought of him struggling to get home while he was still worn out from coming was more than

I could bear. I took a deep breath and astonished everybody.

'I think you'd better come on honeymoon with us,' I said, looking from father to son. They also took deep breaths. Taking a third person on a honeymoon was a novelty that called for deep breaths. The two men stood for a moment looking at each other then my airman beamed and I knew I had done the right thing. It took us a while to persuade his father that I had done the right thing, but when we had the three of us went off on our honeymoon with the others waving frantically from the forecourt of the pub and pelting us with the confetti the vicar had banned.

My mother was delighted to see my father-in-law, for as she said, it gave her a chance to meet him which if we hadn't taken him she never would, what with him living all that way up there and the trains and suchlike.

What she didn't say, but I knew without her saying it, was that having three people spending a honeymoon under her roof rather than the customary two gave her a heaven-sent opportunity to rearrange the sleeping arrangements. She looked ten years younger now that the consummation was having to be postponed through lack of space. She rushed round, airing sheets and blankets, and fixing things so that her new son-in-law shared a room with his father and I tossed and turned on a camp-bed among the evacuees.

When the weekend was over, the three of us walked

up the cart-track and down the lane, refreshed and invigorated from the peaceful holiday we'd had. My father-in-law would remember it for the rest of his life. He had gone into the lane one evening and heard a nightingale singing. He had never heard a nightingale before. It made the honeymoon quite perfect for him, and more so since the rest of his life wasn't to be too long drawn-out.

'Well, what was it like?' asked Davies the first time I saw her after I got back on duty.

'What was what like?' I asked, knowing very well.

'What was the honeymoon like, of course,' she said, peering into my face for signs that might tell her.

'Ecstatic,' I lied. I allowed her to believe the lie for a day or two, then I told her the truth and she laughed so much that the tears poured and she had to excuse herself and rush off to the lavatory. But even she liked the bit about the nightingale.

Our new lodgings were all that we hoped they would be. The landlady was kind and went out of her way to make us comfortable. When my airman came home on a forty-eight-hour pass and brought a lot of washing with him she did the washing and went about with a romantic look on her face. She also threw in cups of tea as she had said she would, though she didn't quite throw them in. She knocked very pointedly on the bedroom door, waited to be told to enter, then when she had entered she stood with the cups in her hand gazing down at us, and hovered while we drank the tea. The curious way she kept looking at us made us think she was perhaps reviving old memories.

The second honeymoon was a great improvement on the first.

Chapter Eighteen

WE WERE QUITE wrong about our landlady. Not about her being kind, she was all that and more; what we were wrong about was in thinking that she needed to bring us a cup of tea on our honeymoon in order to revive old memories. She had no such needs. She lived in the present and not in the past. The present for her was full of exciting adventures brought on by the war. Nance had really only begun to live after the war started. Nance was the name she begged us to call her from the first day we arrived at her house with our few belongings.

Davies was a little sad when I moved from Mrs Darcy's. She had always said that my being married would change everything, notwithstanding the fact that the marriage was more of a part-time luxury than an everyday sameness. She remembered clearly the difference marriage had made to Baker and Weldon. Though they remained our friends there were things in their lives we could no longer share. I soon began to realize that Davies was right. There were things in my life that she could no longer share. One of these was my husband's washing.

For a long time his washing was Nance's responsibility. She had watched me trying to do it one evening after I came off duty and decided that it would be better all round if she gave me a few lessons before letting me loose among the suds. I had never done any washing, beyond the occasional pair of stockings or gloves. I had sometimes been allowed to turn the mangle at home on Mondays but by the time I got up in the morning the whites were already boiling in the copper and the coloureds ready to be scrubbed to a paler shade than they were before. Washday at home had been a day's work, starting at the crack of dawn and finishing with the final bit of ironing almost at bedtime. I had had very little share in it. I needed several lessons from Nance before I learnt the knack of sorting the whites from the coloureds, and even then I often allowed a black sock to stray among the white vests and pants. Luckily my husband was still besotted enough to see his greyish underwear and white-streaked socks through rose-coloured spectacles.

Cooking was another thing that Nance taught me. She said that knowing how to cook might come in handy some day. 'Come in handy' was one of Nance's favourite expressions. She used it often, and in some very peculiar places. She stood one day with a loaf of bread in her hand and a look of wonder on her face. 'I do like to have a bit of bread in the house,' she said dreamily. 'It do come in handy sometimes.' I had to agree that it did.

My mother had taught me as little about cooking as she had about washing. She liked the kitchen to herself, especially on Fridays, which were baking days. She became extremely angry if people like me got under her feet while she was busy with the dough: she said it stopped it rising properly and caused a draught that cooled the oven. I kept well out of the way on baking day. But Nance didn't mind me being under her feet. She showed me how to make cakes, using liquid paraffin instead of rationed margarine; she taught me how to transform uneatable scraps of meat into even less eatable rissoles and she initiated me into the correct way of boiling an egg. Four verses of 'Onward, Christian Soldiers' sung to a slow march tempo would produce an egg firm without being too hard. Lightly boiled would only take three verses. Having sung in the church choir from an early age at home, I was familiar with the words of 'Onward, Christian Soldiers' and could sing them off by heart. It was one of the better uses to which I put my religious education.

Nance also tried to teach me how to make a Yorkshire pudding but she soon gave up. Her way was very different from the way my mother had made them. My mother's were airy-fairy things that rose to a tremendous height, almost touching the top of the oven. Nance's were thick and stodgy, baked in a pie dish and as flat when they came out of the oven as they were when they went in. I had never actually made a Yorkshire pudding but I knew from listening to my mother how they should be made. When my mother beat the batter she beat it for a long time and you could hear the noise right through the house. Nance just stirred it with a spoon. We finally agreed to differ over how a Yorkshire pudding should be made.

But except for this one small difference I owed a great deal to Nance's patient grounding in washing and cooking. Though, despite all her efforts, I never became properly proficient at ironing shirts. The holes where the cuff links should have glided through effortlessly were never positioned in the way they should have been. Putting in a cuff link could take a long time, especially if the shirt had been well starched. Beneath my iron the tail-ends became lake-smooth while the fronts rippled like a puddle in a storm. In one way and another shirts caused me a great deal of trouble.

Just as Andy on Male Surgery had demanded payment for whatever he did for us as a favour, so Nance demanded her pound of flesh in return for her services to me. Some of her demands were out of all proportion to the services rendered. But I paid. She had ways of making me pay.

She was a handsome woman, in her late thirties, she told me once, but secretly I thought forty was nearer the truth. And even that was being kind. She had jet-black hair which she kept jet-black with the regular applications of some kind of lotion. She was blessed with a fashion sense which made me feel very dowdy. Not since Laura, a prosperous prostitute I had nursed a long time ago, invited me to her flat to show me her clothes had I felt so shabby. Nance, like Laura, knew the right thing to wear and, what was more important, seemed to have it to wear. Compared to hers my wardrobe was a paltry thing.

Her husband was an insignificant little man, totally overshadowed by his wife's outstanding attributes. He worshipped her, and not merely for her outstanding attributes. He even worshipped the ground she walked on. He fetched and carried, brought and took, gave her a cup of tea before he went to work in the morning and her breakfast in bed on Sundays. He found aspirins for her migraines and antacid powders for her stomach upsets. He was a good husband. He was exactly the sort of husband the psychiatrist had in mind when he said with professional insight: 'Show me a good husband and I will show you his neurotic wife.'

But Nance kept her neuroses for her husband. While he was around she suffered every complaint she'd heard about in the shops that morning and many more that I told her about while we were sitting on her docket-bought rexine sofa. She came out in spots if he said anything to upset her and retired to her room with the curtains drawn and vinegar cloths if he looked like asking for something she didn't feel like giving him – his conjugal rights, for example. She didn't give him those very often, she told me; it was funny, she said, how she got a bit of a headache the moment she got into bed.

He bore it all with fortitude. She was, he confided in me sadly one day, the victim of her nerves and more to be pitied than blamed. Going without his conjugal rights was a small price to pay for her happiness. He had gone without them so often that the sum must have been considerable.

Because he was a good husband he allowed her more freedom than most wives got before the post-war era started giving them all they wanted. He was the first to admit that she needed a bit of fresh air after a busy day at the ammunition factory where she worked. For a long time he had said nothing when the bit of fresh air was taken in the evening and well on into the night. He had only started asking awkward questions a week or two before I went to live there. I arrived in time to save Nance from a severe restriction of her freedom.

I got in from the hospital one evening to find her looking breathtaking in a sequined gown, a pair of spindly silver shoes, and her hair cascading down her back with a few extra sequins scattered amongst it. Her husband was in his working clothes. He was hopping about doing up buttons and fastening beads.

His face shone with pride at the radiance of the woman he had married. She accepted his homage as her due.

During a brief moment while he rushed upstairs to exchange the gold mesh bag that matched nothing for the silver one to go with her shoes she told me what I had to do in return for all she had done for me. I listened intently.

First, she said, I had to stay up instead of having the early night I'd been looking forward to while I was puffing home on my bike. Then, having stayed up, I was to sit on the sofa and keep her husband's mind off the fact that she wasn't there. Lately, she said, he'd started worrying a bit about the nights out she was having with the girls from the factory. One a week he could understand, but two struck him as a bit excessive, however close the friendship was with the girls. It was my job, said Nance, to persuade him that sequins and silver and two nights out a week were a necessary part of the social life at the factory. Once he was persuaded and had gone off to bed I was to stay awake until I heard her throwing stones at my window, then I was to creep down quietly and let her in. Staying up to let her in was another thing her husband had started getting funny about lately, she said.

I did all she asked. The American airmen who brought her to the door were far better looking than the girls from the factory.

Davies was very shocked when I told her what I was having to do to keep my landlady happy. She said she didn't think it was fair on the husband. I could see her point but, as I told her, I would have done just the same for him if he'd asked me. He never did. He was quite content to stay in every night, listening to the wireless and talking to me about the absent one. He never had been one for going out much, he told me. I thought that was a pity. With a wife like Nance it might have been better to have kept up with her occasionally.

When Nance kindly invited me to make a foursome with her, her current boyfriend and my new husband I was very excited about it. She told me that we would go to London in a hired car, have a bite to eat somewhere and go to a show. She promised to lend me a few of her sequins to pep up my wedding dress and give it more of the party spirit. At the last minute my airman had his leave stopped. He wrote and said how sorry he was and he hoped I would still go, it seemed a pity not to when Nance had been kind enough to invite me. I told her I would go and she arranged with her current boyfriend to bring a friend for me. She stressed that he had to be married so that I would know there was nothing to get worried about. She pinned a few artificial flowers on the bodice of my wedding dress, lent me a string of pearls with earrings to match and we waited for our escorts. Nance's husband had been told the truth about the night out in London, since my going as well lent a respectability to the outing which cast out any doubts he might have had when the Americans rolled up at the door.

The hired car we drove off in, leaving Nance's husband waving on the doorstep, was very grand. I sank into the back seat beside the boyfriend's best friend and Nance sat in front being the life and soul of the party. She sounded very vivacious. Her husband wouldn't have known her. Gone was the migraine, banished the biliousness.

Her boyfriend seemed to know London well. Far better than many Londoners. He drove us straight to a garage in the middle of somewhere where the oldest profession in the world prospered and flourished. There were 'Lauras' everywhere. The only difference I could see between these 'Lauras' and the Laura I had treated at the special clinic for so long was that these girls looked even more prosperous; but that was probably because though the cost of living was higher in London the wages of sin were more inflated.

When the car was safely garaged we walked through several small and busy streets. The business being done on the pavements involved some haggling between client and operator over rates for the job.

The theatre on a corner that we eventually arrived at looked very small. I had never been to a theatre before. I thought of *Romeo and Juliet* and a few Greek tragedies I had read at school but one look at the posters that covered the walls told me that it was none of these I was about to see. The girls on the posters wore fewer clothes than Juliet and the few they wore were certainly not Grecian. There was a long queue outside the theatre, mostly of servicemen. One or two had their girlfriends with them but only one or two. I began to feel very conspicuous. Nance appeared to be taking it all in her stride.

The lady who sat in the ticket office when we finally reached the head of the queue was the soul of respectability. She wore a black gown of impeccable taste and three rows of pearls. She could have been Mrs Darcy's sister.

The girl who came round selling programmes wore neither a black gown nor any pearls. She wasn't wearing much of anything. She had a few feathers arranged in places where the arrangement mattered most and she sold her programmes as if she was handing out favours. Our escorts paid eagerly for her favours.

Beyond a muttered thank you for the ice cream that one of the men bought me during the interval I sat through the whole show without saying a word. The girls on the stage had changed from feathers to fans and the fans were no more successful at concealment than the feathers. However carefully they were manipulated they still left enough open spaces to send the men whistling like a boiling kettle.

When some motionless nudes started posing on plinths the men were first stunned to silence, then awakened to thunderous ecstasy. They forgot for a while the war they had left outside, and the fighting they would be going back to when their leave was over. The memory of the nudes would perhaps make the fighting easier to bear. Later, we heard that the sirens had gone while we were in the theatre but since it hadn't closed even for the Blitz it was hardly likely to panic over a stray bomber that might only have been passing over London on its way to somewhere else.

The two men led Nance and me back through the dark streets and to a tiny restaurant that you wouldn't have known was a restaurant unless somebody had recommended it to you. Somebody had obviously recommended it to the two Americans. It was so dimly lit that we could scarcely see what we were eating. Not that it mattered. The food tasted so awful that seeing it could only have made matters worse. The men weren't interested in what they were eating. They were more interested in the girls who fluttered in the candlelight like gauzy moths. Though the cost of the meal had to be kept down to five shillings there were various temptations put in the men's way to induce them to spend more. Among the inducements were tiny fluffy dolls, the exact replicas of the girls who were twirling the men's hair round their fingers. The fluff on the dolls matched the fluff on the girls, and they even had matching diamonds stuck to their navels. The men bought Nance and me a doll each.

It was very late when we left the restaurant. We walked slowly back to the garage. The street trade had thinned out a bit and Nance and I stood on the pavement and waited while the men went across for the car. We had been standing for a few minutes when an attendant from the garage rushed across the road, grabbed the two of us and hustled us over to the garage. He was quite out of breath with hurrying.

'I shouldn't stand there if I were you, Miss,' he said, looking at Nance. 'It might start giving the reg'lars ideas. We don't want them getting ideas, do we, Miss?' Nance agreed that giving the reg'lars ideas might not be at all wise. The man said something about getting your faces slashed with a razor and Nance pressed twopence into his hand. I couldn't help thinking that one look at my wedding dress and navy blue mac would dispel any ideas the reg'lars might have had of competition from me. Though Nance's sequins might just have triggered something off.

When we reached home we said a quick goodnight and thank you to the men then hammered on the door to be let in.

I didn't say anything to Davies about the theatre or the restaurant. I fobbed her off with a few innocent things which appeared to satisfy her. I threw away the fluffy doll before my husband came home on his next leave. Seeing it lying around would have made him ask even more questions about the night out than he did ask. I went into no details about the theatre and I didn't breathe a word about the fans and feathers. I was afraid he might suggest we went there some time. And I really couldn't have borne to stand in the queue again, nor eat the dreadful food in the restaurant. So I kept quiet about it.

Chapter Nineteen

D-DAY CAME AND went, and because it was such a glorious victory after all the defeats we'd been hearing about, some of us were deluded into thinking that the war might almost be over. We were wrong to have such stupid thoughts. There was still more to come.

When the flying bomb landed on the town we felt we had been grossly misled. We couldn't believe that after all this time we had been chosen for one final grand fling by the enemy. Later, when we went down and looked at the chaos the bomb had brought, we marvelled that the people in the big cities had endured what they had endured for so long without going to pieces with fear and horror. Many of them had, but the great majority hadn't. It was the same in our town.

The bang came in the middle of the morning. The patients instinctively dived down their beds, then came up again looking shamefaced at being so silly when the bang could only possibly have been a sudden loud clap of thunder almost over their heads. We were still teasing them about it when we were told to get beds ready for casualties. We had to take one of the girls over to Male Surgery in a wheelchair to sit by her brother's bed until he died. We all felt worse about him dying than we might have felt if he had died while everybody else was dying.

Davies told me that the parents of the child who died on her ward refused to believe it. They had gone so long with nothing too terrible happening that to be robbed of all they held dear when the war was supposed to be over had to be a lie. But it wasn't. Soon more flying bombs were falling and more casualties fell, to be brought into us if bringing them into us had any point to it. The mini-Blitz that the flying bombs brought kept nurses busy until the bases from where they were sent had been destroyed.

The flying bombs were jokingly nicknamed doodle-bugs and buzz-bombs, but they were no joke at all to the people they either merely terrified or sadly maimed. The distant hum of a buzz-bomb could keep us rooted to the spot in petrified anticipation, waiting for the humming to stop. When it did was the time to run for cover. The bang was due at any moment.

Things soon became as if another war had broken out. But this small war was badly resented. It had come too late. All the fun had gone out of the blackout and only despair was left. But very soon even the flying bombs and rockets became commonplace. The more intrepid stood at street corners watching the fierce flames shooting out of the back of a rocket with as much fascination as they would have watched an unidentified flying object had such been on the scene in those days.

Davies didn't like the new missiles at all, but there was soon something to take her mind off them for at least a short time.

She had begged me to go back with her to Mrs Darcy's one evening, instead of going straight back to Nance's. Despite the flying bombs and her dread of them she was beginning at last to look into the future. The rumours of some sort of victory had brought Archibald a little nearer for her. His letters had an underlying hopefulness and while she was reading them her face lost a little of its sadness. Whatever the prison camp had done to him she was prepared for it and ready to nurse him with love until it was all forgotten. It was never quite all forgotten. It would need a lot of time and a lot of love to eradicate some of the worst memories, but Davies was a patient and loving girl.

'I've got something to tell you,' she said mysteriously as we crept into Mrs Darcy's front door and up the stairs. Like Mary the home-sister, Mrs Darcy didn't encourage her residents to have non-resident visitors. There were no evacuees left in the servants' quarters. One by one they had gone, taking their children with them. The lull between the big bombs and the smaller flying ones had made them think it would be safe to go home. For some of the evacuees it hadn't been safe at all. If a flying bomb missed them there was still a rocket to come and get them.

I looked round at the antique grandeur of Davies's bedroom and compared it with the matchstick impermanence of the room I slept in at Nance's. I flicked my ash in the rose-sprigged chamberpot under Davies's bed. There were no such conveniences where I lived. Nance would have been shocked at the very idea. Even Mrs Darcy's chamberpots were soon to be snapped up by Americans at inflated prices to be taken back home as souvenirs. Nance did acquire one much later, but she put a pot plant in it and kept it in the hall. By being in the hall instead of under a bed it gained a lot of respectability.

'I'm going to be a sister,' said Davies breathlessly. I stared at her. We had been staff-nurses for so long it had never occurred to me that we could someday be sisters.

'How long have you known?' I asked.

'Only since this morning,' said Davies. 'The Matron sent for me and told me. She said I can start at the beginning of next month.' I felt no envy that Davies was suddenly to become senior to me even though she had started her training only three months before me. She had all the qualities that would make her a good sister, and a kind one as well.

'There's something I've got to show you,' said Davies. 'Shut your eyes and don't look.' I shut my eyes. I could hear her crashing round the room, pulling out drawers and flinging open doors. After a while there was silence.

'You can look now,' said Davies. I opened my eyes and there she was – Sister Davies.

The uniform didn't quite fit her. The dress was too long and the apron too short, but the frilly lacy cap sat well on her dark hair.

I did a few quick alterations to the dress and apron then sat back to admire the finished product. I was happy for Davies. She was a born nurse and deserved all she got. I just hoped I wouldn't have to be the staff-nurse on her ward. The memories of our training days were still too vivid suddenly to turn us into different grades. She would only have to get cross with me for something and we would both remember our early training and how she rescued me from drowning in the sluice when I had turned on a wrong tap. I would need all my carefully trained respect for my seniors to be able to keep a straight face.

Soon there were things to take my mind off Davies and her new status. It was on the day that Nance's niece got married that I started to make some interesting discoveries about a possible new status for myself.

It had been hoped that Nance's niece would have the wedding over and done with before her shape proclaimed to the world that the honeymoon was a thing of the past. But in the way of many wartime weddings nothing had gone according to plan and by the time everything, except the baby, had been arranged in its proper sequence a bed was already booked for Nance's niece in the local maternity hospital.

On the morning of the wedding I got up early to give Nance a hand with the catering. I had asked for a day off for the occasion. The reception was being held in Nance's front room. She was giving it to the bride as a wedding present.

We were halfway through the bloater paste sandwiches when I had a sudden feeling that if I saw another bit of bloater paste I wouldn't be responsible for my stomach. I asked Nance whether she would mind if I left them to her and went on to arranging the cup cakes. Nance was a dab hand at cup cakes. She gave me a sharp look and moved over. And my stomach settled down.

Nance's niece was a popular girl, liked by all who knew her. Partly because of her popularity, and partly because everybody expected her to have the baby on the altar steps, the church was packed. It was standing room only in all parts and a three-deep queue out in the churchyard.

Nance had managed to beg, borrow, or barter enough clothing coupons to ensure that her niece would stagger up the aisle radiantly beautiful in a snowy white, all-enveloping gown, with demure brides-maids and bashful pageboys in attendance, all looking as sweetly innocent as the bride did.

To Nance's relief and everybody else's disappointment the baby held off until its expectant parents were in the room overlooking the sea, where they had gone for a short, and second, honeymoon. Then the excitement became too much for it and a midwife had to be sent for in a hurry.

The excitement had been too much for me as well. When the last guest had gone and Nance's husband had done the washing-up we left him to tidy the front room while we went into the kitchen and had a cup of tea. It was while we were drinking the tea that Nance peered into my face.

'You're looking a bit off-colour, dear,' she said. 'Aren't you feeling yourself?' I realized when she said it that I hadn't felt myself for several days, particularly in the morning. Until then I had always felt myself in the morning.

'Have a fag,' said Nance. I shrank away from the cigarette she was offering me and she gave me another close look. After years of smoking all the cigarettes I could afford the thought of one more did the same to my stomach as the bloater paste had.

'Gone off fags as well then, have we?' I nodded, feeling suddenly sorry for myself. The tears welled up in my eyes.

'There's nothing to fret about,' said Nance briskly. 'You're expecting, that's all.' And so I was.

After I had written a letter telling my husband he was going to be a father, and another to my mother telling her she was going to be a grandmother I plucked up courage and went to tell the Matron that I was expecting to become a mother. She wasn't nearly as enchanted about it as my husband and my mother had been. I was very glad I hadn't made any rash promises when I was asking her if I could get married. She would certainly have cast it up at me. Getting married didn't necessarily rob the hospital of a nurse, but having a baby most certainly did.

'And when is the event due to take place?' the Matron asked, after she had recovered a little from the bad news. I did a quick bit of calculation based on Nance's informed forecasting, and assured her that I was good for another three or four months' work. She seemed vastly relieved and sent me back to work on the Male ward where I was currently employed.

It wasn't long before the patients were using their powers of observation on me as keenly as I had used mine on them through the years. They became embarrassingly interested in my interesting condition. It also had its lighter moments for them.

The top of the pops song that was being plugged by the disc jockeys of the day was called 'I Got Spurs that Jingle Jangle Jingle'. Long before the spurs were through their jingling I was going at top speed up the ward, looking for somewhere private to leave my breakfast. The smell of roasting chestnuts had the same effect on me.

Outside one of the ward windows there was an enormous sweet chestnut tree. From the day the annexes were built the patients on them who were able to walk walked out when the sister's back was turned and collected the chestnuts to roast on top of the red-hot coke stove. I still dislike the smell of roasting chestnuts.

When the sister on the men's ward grew tired of seeing my rapidly increasing girth squeezing between lockers and through doors she sent me back to the Matron. This time even she could see that there was nothing she could do to stem the tide of nature, but instead of suggesting that I should leave and spend my waiting days with my feet up in Nance's front room she made me go to the children's block until I had worked my month's notice. Fortunately for me the sister was married; she was happily aware that it could be her turn to get a funny tummy when something didn't suit it so she let me sit in the ward kitchen, sipping soda water where there were no jangling spurs to ruin the day for me.

At the end of the month I walked down the road to my lodgings. As I walked a siren went, nobody took any notice of it and it was soon followed by the All Clear. At last the war was receding into the background. I turned the corner and stopped for a moment, looking back at the hospital. Foolishly I thought that my nursing days were over.

I was very much mistaken.

About the Author

Brought up in Lincolnshire, Evelyn Prentis (real name Evelyn Taws) left home at eighteen to become a nurse. She later moved to London during the war, where she married and raised her family. Like so many other nurses, she went back to hospital and used any spare time she might have had bringing up her children and running her home. Born in 1915, she sadly died in 2001 at the age of eighty-five.

Evelyn published five books about her life as a nurse, and Ebury Press are reissuing them all. *A Nurse in Time* and *A Nurse in Action* are the first two, and *A Nurse and Mother* will follow shortly.

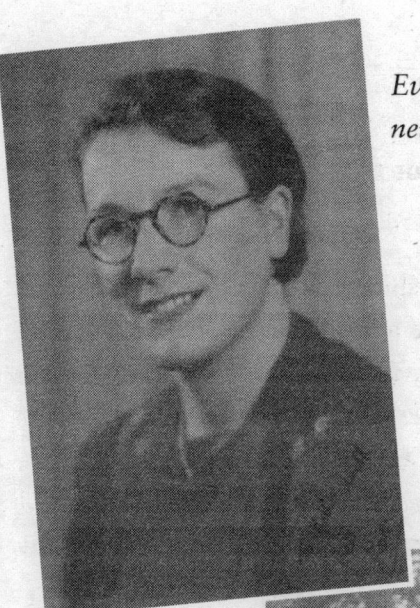

Evelyn Prentis in 1938, newly qualified

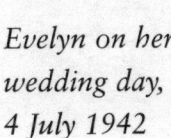

Evelyn on her wedding day, 4 July 1942